DOC-RELATED

2022

**A Physician's Guide To
Fixing Our Ailing Health Care System**

Contents

Introduction

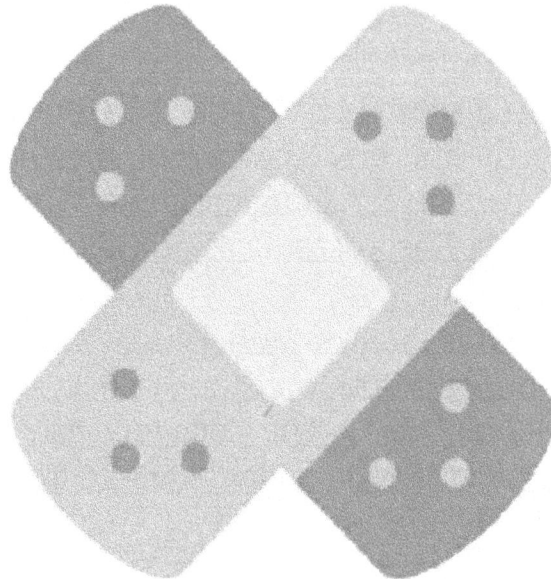

Health care is the largest employer in the United States (U.S.), with over 16 million people in the industry. Over one million of them are practicing physicians. I'm one of them. Nearly 70 percent of physicians are employed by hospitals or corporate entities. Corporate entities include health insurers, private equity firms, and entities that own multiple physician practices.

For physicians, rising practice costs and stagnant reimbursements have made it difficult to be independent. Doctors also see the writing on the wall related to emerging payment models that will require large financial investments in care management and information technology. In addition, the physician workforce is getting younger, and they desire more work-life balance, not the long hours I practiced earlier in my career. The result is that healthcare professionals are sacrificing full autonomy for stability.

When I began practicing in 2001, I was the medical director of a rural clinic in Texas, performing the full scope of family medicine, including clinic, inpatient care, emergency room, nursing home, and even home visits. I delivered babies, performed c-sections, endoscopies, tubal ligations, tonsillectomies and assisted with various other surgeries. I followed my patients and their families throughout the continuum of care.

Back then, I worked endless hours, but always loved what I did. That was a time before electronic health records and other programs and regulations increased the workload of what we do today. I'm not trying to argue against these measures, but they have taken a toll on the joy of practicing medicine.

While practicing rural medicine, I realized I knew little about the business side of medicine, so I went back to school to get my Master of Business Administration (MBA). The business degree gave me new insights on streamlining workflows, health care finance, and how our system compares to other developed countries. It ignited a passion for me to change the industry on a bigger scale.

As I've transitioned from full-time clinical care to more administrative responsibilities, it's been eye-opening to see how organizations make strategic and financial decisions. Research shows that only 16 percent of health care organizations consider the impact of strategic decisions on the resilience and well-being of those affected. I initially thought writing about the inefficiencies in our health care system and its impact on health care professionals would be dated. That organizations would have solved this problem. Unfortunately, not much has changed over the last few years.

I've always had a sense of humor about health care. This became official when my classmates named me class comedian in medical school. Malcolm Gladwell said, "Comedians have become the truth tellers. Satire allows you to say almost anything. That's where truth is spoken to power in our society. When you sugar-coat a bitter truth with humor, it makes the medicine go down."

It was as I continuously encountered physician dissatisfaction and organizational dysfunction that the idea for Doc-Related was born. I love to draw, and I wanted to apply satire to raise awareness about organizational disconnects. The more I thought about it, the more the characters for a comic strip took shape in my head. The comics have been therapeutic for me, inspired by actual events occurring within care centers across America today.

My twenty-year career has taken me from practicing rural medicine, to academics, to multi-specialty medical groups, to integrated delivery networks. In that time, I've had the fortune, or maybe misfortune, to experience both sides of the table. I continue to practice part-time as a family physician, and I work as an executive with oversight of large multi-specialty medical groups. My focus as a doctor and as a leader has always been to provide patients with the best care possible while making sure our health care professionals and staff feel valued and appreciated for their efforts.

This book is a medley of anecdotes and comics supported with timely data presented in a satirical format. The chapters identify what's broken in our health care system for patients, physicians and practice leaders, along with what we can do to fix them.

Section one targets the human aspects of expectations and behaviors, including (1) patient surveys, (2) leadership and communication, (3) staff support, and operations. The second section covers how health care providers are paid and what affects payments including (4) insurance, (5) coding, (6) prior authorizations, and (7) measuring productivity. Section three addresses charting and regulatory challenges, including (8) dealing with electronic health records (EHR), (9) tracking metrics and (10) dealing with malpractice.

My goal is to highlight not only how our ailing health care system affects patients, but how it affects those seeking to provide the care — and ways we can make it better. Whether you work in the health care field or have had experiences accessing care, this book promises to be entertaining and informative.

Part 1:
Human Dynamics

Chapter 1
The Changing Landscape: Meet the Crew

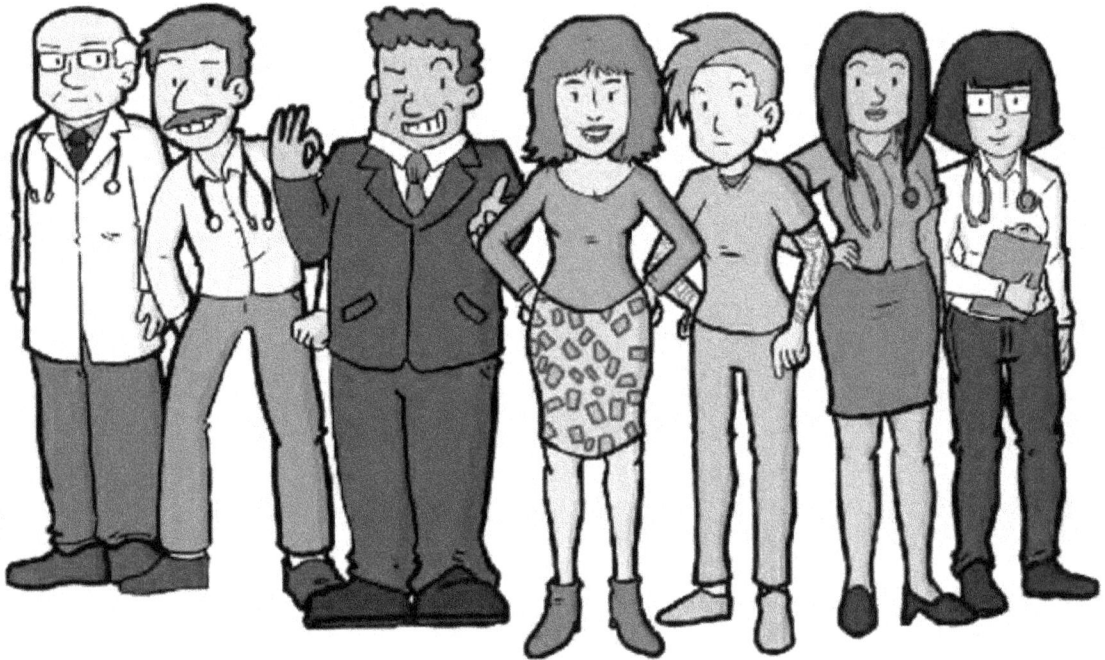

Like all industries, today's health care workplace brings together several generational cohorts. This includes Boomers, early to mid-career Xers, and Millennials. Each is unique in their motivations, communication style, and worldview. Research from the Pew Institute describes Baby Boomers aka Boomers (born between 1946-1964) as competitive, workaholic, and team oriented. Company loyalty and duty motivate them. They prefer communicating via phone calls and face-to-face and enjoy being involved in work decisions. Their view of the world is that people must pay their dues and sacrifice to achieve success. Boomers currently comprise 25% of the U.S. workforce.

Generation Xers (born between 1965-1980) are more casual, skeptical, and independent. Diversity, work-life balance, and their own personal interest over that of the company motivate them. Their communication preference is like Boomers via face-to-face and phone calls, but they're not objectionable to emails or texts. Their view of the world depends on its impact on them directly. Gen Xers can be resistant to change at work if it affects their personal lives. They comprise 33% of the labor force in the U.S.

Millennials (born 1981–2000) are achievement-oriented and civic-minded. Unique work experiences motivate them, and they prefer to communicate via texts, instant messaging, and email. They base their view of the world on personal growth and development, having work-life balance, and fun at work. Like Gen Xers, Millennials don't necessarily share company loyalty and may leave an organization if they don't like change. They comprise 35% of the U.S. Workforce, and approximately 15% still live at home with their parents.

What's most important to understand is that employers should not treat all staff the same and expect the same outcomes. During my career, I've had Boomer clinicians call me "wet behind the ears," and Millennial clinicians tell me they appreciate my leadership style because I'm never "salty." I knew wet behind the ears referred to my age and inexperience, but I had to look up salty. For those of you not hip to the slang, it means being in a foul mood, bitter, or harboring grudges.

I must admit, I've been looking up millennial terms more often than ever since I ended a group email with "stay thirsty," thinking it would be cool to reference the Most Interesting Man in the World from Dos Equis commercials while encouraging others to hunger for knowledge and curiosity. I found out later that in millennial terms, "thirsty" refers to hungering for attention, being needy, or desperate.

Some people might argue that categorizing people based on their age is like thinking you know someone based on his or her astrology sign. However, there are similarities in people based on world events that have shaped their life. Time will only tell what COVID-19 will do for Generation Z — those born between 1995-2015.

On a lighter note, understanding and dealing with multiple generations in the workforce can be a minefield for managers, but also provides excellent fodder for my comic strips. The characters may even sound familiar. I enjoy having people ask me if I base my characters on actual people because they personify someone they work with or know in health care. The comic strip is not about stereotypes or ageism. It's about characters I've met in my career path.

People also ask if I ever worked in their office because they've experienced one of my comics at their job. It's a testament to the commonality of challenges being seen across the country. Like many industries, my comics incorporate the friction that exists between management and employees. In health care, this friction can be stronger since both sides have higher levels of education and training than other industries, but neither seems to understand the other's challenges. I will cover this more in chapter two.

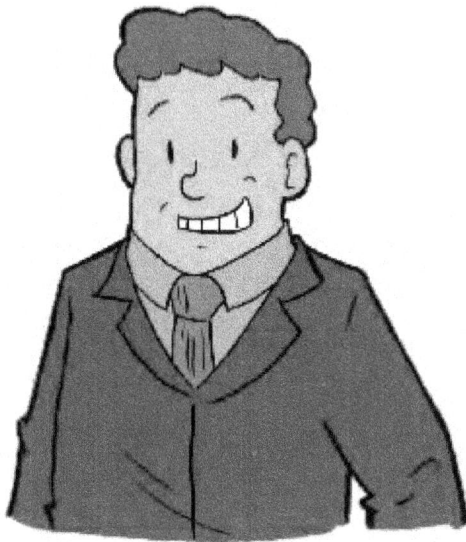

Chip Conner- Vice-President of Operations

Chip is a Gen Xer with a salesman-like approach to solving problems. Although he thinks all docs are his friends and calls them by their first names, they don't trust a word that comes out of his mouth.

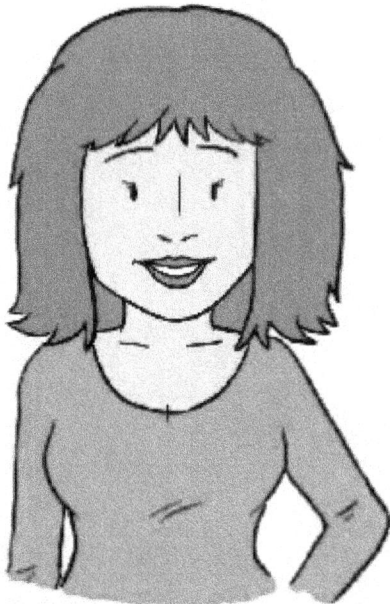

Donna Bloomfield- Clinic Director

Donna reports to Chip. The docs think she does an "okay" job but get frustrated with her inability to provide resources. Donna is a gen-Xer who loves her two cats and wearing leopard-patterned clothing.

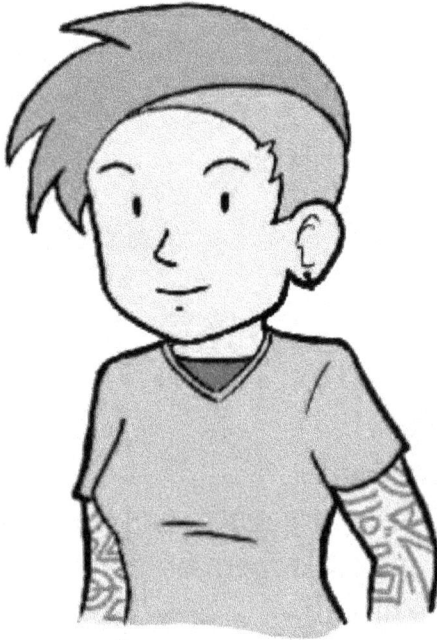

Karla Vitallia- Medical Assistant

Karla is a millennial, relatively new to her role. Her real passions are body art, microbreweries and going on motorcycle cruises with her boyfriend. She's a quick learner and gets along with all the docs.

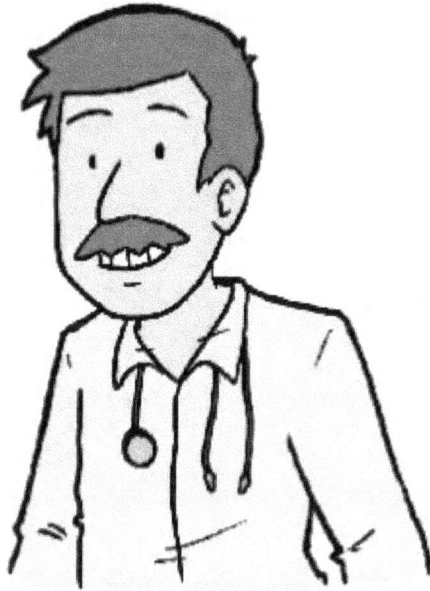

Dr. Tom Stevens- Medical Director

Dr. Stevens is a gen-Xer with an MBA and has a knack for seeing where things are headed. He's well liked and trusted by both the administration and physicians. He gets impatient at times with how slow things move.

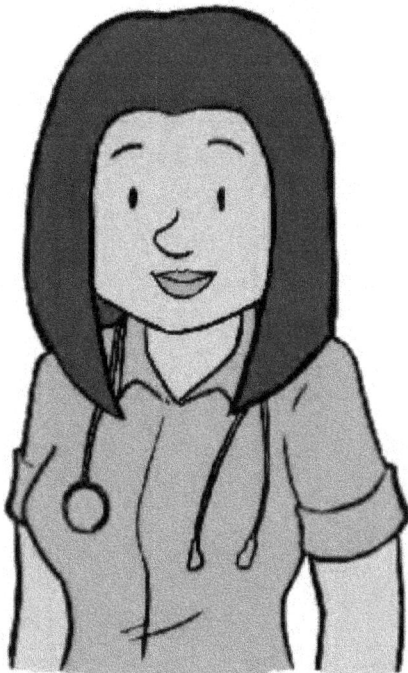

Dr. Anika Shah- Clinic Physician

Dr. Shah is a millennial physician whose major focus is getting home to her husband and twin toddlers at a decent hour. She's been in practice for 5 years and enjoys personal fitness and fashion.

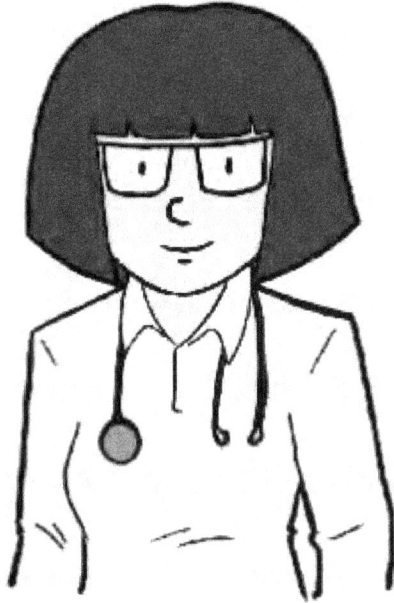

Dr. Cici Lam- Clinic Physician

Dr. Lam is a millennial physician who recently joined the group. She's fresh out of residency and still has much to learn about the bureaucracies of practicing medicine. Cici is single and enjoys spending time reading and surfing the internet.

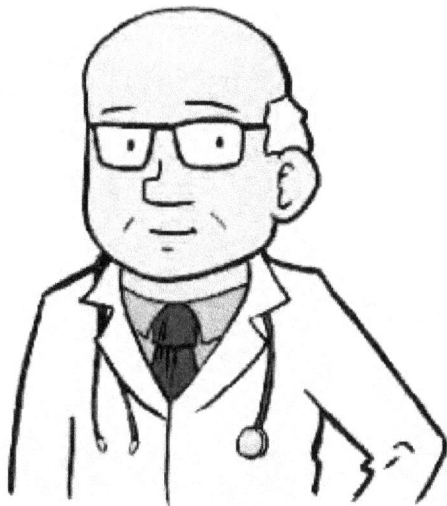

Dr. Harold Katz- Clinic Physician

Dr. Katz is a baby boomer at the end of his career. He was in private practice for over 30 years before his practice was acquired by the group. He's not a big fan of anything corporate and is nostalgic for the old ways of practicing medicine using pen and paper.

Chapter 2
Patient Surveys: The Quest for Positive Reviews

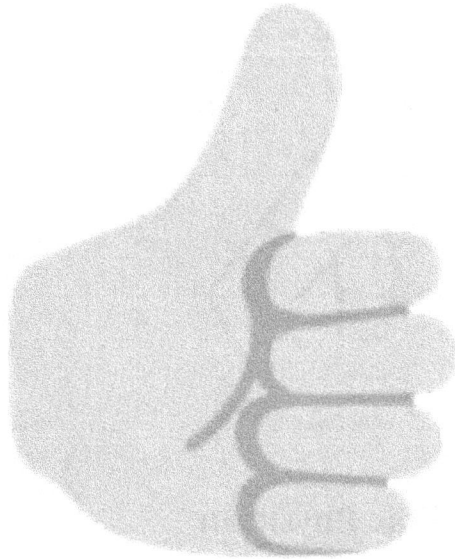

Early in my career as a rural physician in Texas, I took care of a couple in their mid-70s named Vernon and Nellie. They drove in from another small town 50 miles away. Nellie usually did all the talking, while her husband, Vernon, sat quietly next to her.

Each visit, she would tell me how Vernon had endangered his health. "Dr. Valenzuela, Vernon ate ice cream for lunch, and I told him that was bad for his sugar diabetes. Dr. Valenzuela, Vernon ate popcorn last night, and I told him that was gonna make his blood pressure worse. Dr. Valenzuela, Vernon just won't listen to me when I tell him he's gonna end up deader than a doornail." As she spoke, Vernon would just roll his eyes, tilt his head down and slump in his chair.

Each time I tried to engage Vernon about his health, he could only get a few words out before Nellie interrupted. I sympathized with the guy, but he refused to see me alone. Vernon was a Korean War veteran with PTSD, who hated clinics and hospitals.

One day, Nellie walked into the exam room in high spirits. I could tell she had some big news for me, so I obliged and said, "My goodness Nellie, I've never seen you glowing as much as you are today. What's the occasion?" She smiled from ear-to-ear and said, "Dr. Valenzuela, Vernon and I just celebrated our 50-year wedding anniversary! Can you believe we've been married for 50 years?"

Vernon piped up and said, "Dr. Valenzuela, I know it's been 50 years, but I swear it feels like five minutes." Just as I was about to compliment Vernon for being so romantic, he leans forward in his chair and finishes with "… under water. Five minutes under water!" My first response was to just about to fall out of my chair laughing as I watched a rare grin on Vernon's face. Nellie's ear-to-ear smile twisted into a scowl. Nellie responded by saying, "He's always trying to be funny, even when he ain't."

It was then that I learned Vernon had a sense of humor and loved to tell jokes, which I viewed as my connection with him. From that point on, I'd be sure to ask Vernon if he'd heard any good jokes during each visit. He always had a new one for me, although not all of them were for general consumption. Appealing to Vernon's sense of humor actually made him more compliant with his medical conditions, although he still cheated on his diet from time to time.

Back then, my visits with Vernon and Nellie lasted an hour by the time we'd addressed his multitude of chronic conditions, saw new photos of the grandkids, and talked about social events at the Veterans of Foreign Wars (VFW) hall. I'd like to think they enjoyed having me as a physician, but those were the days before we measured patient satisfaction. Back when docs didn't get feedback through the Clinician and Group Consumer Assessment of Healthcare Providers and Systems (CG-CAHPS) or Yelp. The only way we knew if our patients were happy with our services was when they verbalized it. From time to time — particularly during the holidays — we also received gifts from grateful patients. The gifts were commonly food or treats to share will all the staff. Today, we use surveys to better understand and improve our patients' experiences with health care providers and staff.

Statistically, it's likely that Vernon and Nellie would have scored me high on patient experience surveys, not because I was an exceptional doctor, but because older, sicker patients who generate higher health care costs rate their providers better . On the downside, as a new physician still establishing my practice in a rural area, other patients would have likely scored me lower simply because expectations and demands are different for new physicians with whom they haven't established a relationship.

Patient Experience Versus Patient Satisfaction

To complicate matters, clinicians are being rated and scored based on patient experience AND patient satisfaction. Although used interchangeably, they're not the same thing. To measure patient experience, we have to ask patients whether something that should happen in a health care setting actually happened. They target what happened. The questions are standardized to be objective. For example, "Did you see the physician within 15 minutes of your scheduled appointment?" Patient satisfaction deals with whether a health encounter met a patient's expectations. In other words, "How did we do?" It's more subjective. An example of patient satisfaction could be whether the patient thought finding parking was a challenge.

CG-CAHPS targets patient experience. Here's why it so important: insurers track CG-CAHPs as a way of monitoring and rewarding health care organizations. As a result, organizations reward, or penalize, physicians based on survey results. Although patient experience surveys are standardized, they are not perfect. Survey findings can vary with how they are administered (phone vs. mail vs. email) and when they are completed (immediately after visit vs. weeks later). The surveys also need a minimum threshold of responses to be statistically significant. The average acceptable sample size is at least 40 responses.

Also, since most physicians score well overall, the clustering for percentile ranking nationally is very close. A CG-CAHPs raw percentage score of 85% (out of 100) for "How Well Providers Communicate with Patients" is only at the 50th percentile, where a raw score of 92—only 7 points higher—places clinicians at the 90th percentile in the nation.

Online physician reviews and ratings target patient satisfaction. As previously noted, this is a more subjective measure. Two people who receive the same care but who have different expectations for how that care should be delivered can give different satisfaction ratings because of their different expectations. Studies show that those physicians with negative online reviews were more often scored poorly due to non-physician specific causes. In my career, I've read comments from patients that said they were not satisfied with their provider because they didn't like the color of the walls in the exam room. Another mentioned that tea wasn't offered in the waiting room, just coffee.

Surveys are not necessarily bad, but they have changed the way we interact with patients. Doctors are now feeling pressured to provide care patients don't need because of fears of bad patient satisfaction scores or negative reviews online. This causes more stress on health care professionals. In a national study, 78% of clinicians said patient satisfaction scores moderately or severely affected their job satisfaction negatively, and 28 percent said the scores made them consider quitting.

Dealing with the Yelp Effect

Measuring and reporting on patient satisfaction within health care has become a major industry. In fact, a recent Google search for "patient satisfaction" reveals 164 MILLION results! To educate the public on how online ratings like Yelp affect physicians and impact patient care, Dr. Zubin Damania, aka ZDoggMD, created a funny, yet sobering musical parody called "Blank Script" based on Taylor Swift's "Blank Space" song about a patient who 'doctor shops' for narcotic medications and threatens to "screw them on Yelp" if they don't abide by their wishes. Uploaded in January 2015, the video has been viewed close to one million times on YouTube.

Besides overprescribing, spending too much time focusing on what patients want may mean they get less of what they really need. Researchers at UC Davis found that the most satisfied patients spent the most on health care. They were 12% more likely to be admitted to the hospital and accounted for 9% more in total health care costs. Even more alarming, they were also the ones more likely to die.

The results could reflect those doctors reimbursed according to patient satisfaction scores may be less inclined to talk patients out of treatments they request or to raise concerns about smoking, substance abuse, or mental-health issues. What makes Yelp and other physician review sites so frustrating is that health care professionals can be disappointed to do an online search of themselves and find random negative reviews or some other misinformation about an experience. In most of these circumstances, physicians are not able to explain themselves or push back on the inaccuracies.

In fact, the Health Insurance Portability and Accountability Act (HIPAA) forbids healthcare providers from responding specifically to a negative review without patient permission. HIPAA is a federal law passed in 1996 requiring the development of national standards to protect sensitive patient health information from being disclosed without the patient's consent or knowledge. Responding to negative reviews is even more challenging in employed models, where organizations have marketing and social media administrators responsible for responding to them. The response is usually generic and only a few sentences.

Ways to Fix How We Use Surveys

The goal of customer surveys is to improve the customer experience. Like any industry, health care should value input from those who pay for and use their services. It should also do its best to make all stakeholders happy with the care they provide. Ideally, this should be based on objective feedback within the control of those providing the care.

Because services provided in the health care industry can lead to bodily harm, the focus of patient surveys in health care should not be to satisfy every patient's expectation of care, but to find ways to improve care. This means treating patients as a partner in producing healthy outcomes.

To curtail the subjectivity of online reviews, vendors should ask standard questions that align with CG-CAHPS surveys. Online patient review sites should also be required to have a minimal sample size of 40-50 responses before posting ratings on any clinician. Given the sensitive nature of the health are industry, they should also establish a review and appeal process prior to posting feedback.

To truly improve care, we should rely on more information than just feedback from patients. Other sources of feedback should include focus groups and patient family advisors. We can also incorporate workplace data like staff surveys. Service data like phone answering rates and turnaround times for patient messages are also vital to care. Administrators should also be involved in helping to improve services through rounding and noting observations at the care centers.

Once we have enough useful information from various sources, we can use the results to improve services in a focused way. William Deming, the father of total quality management, once said, "Eighty-five percent of the reasons for failure are deficiencies in the systems and process rather than the employee. The role of management is to change the process rather than badgering individuals to do better." It's no different in health care.

With this in mind, we should not be rewarding, or penalizing physicians based solely on individual scores. Clinicians should be engaged in making improvements in their care centers, but they should not be solely responsible for patient satisfaction results. Instead, we need to look at entire care teams to enhance care. In the end, by improving the way we provide care, we will positively impact the way patients experience the care they receive.

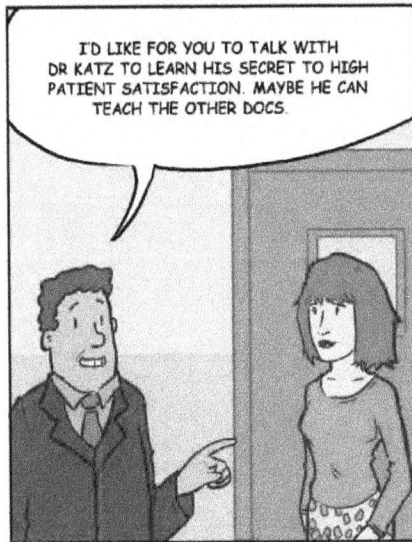

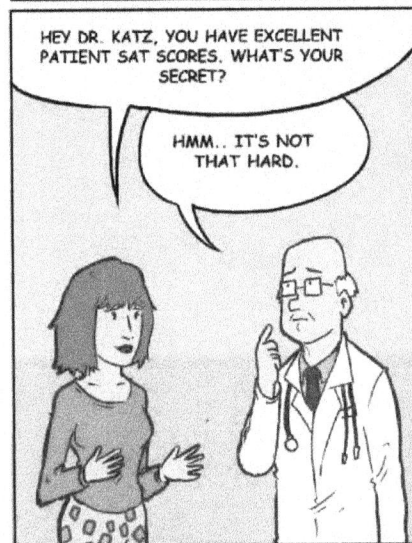

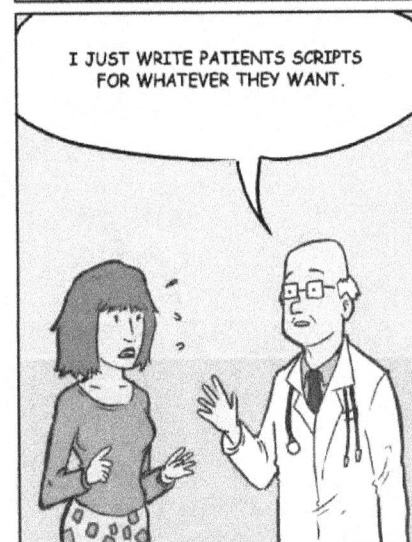

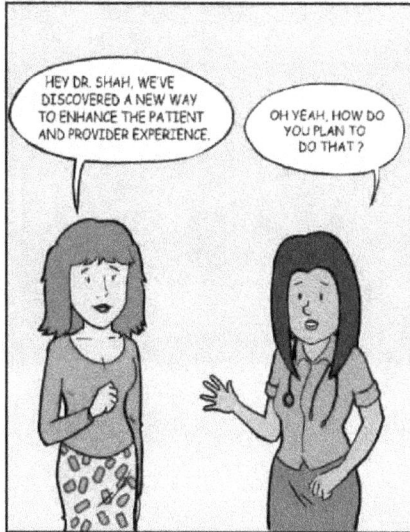

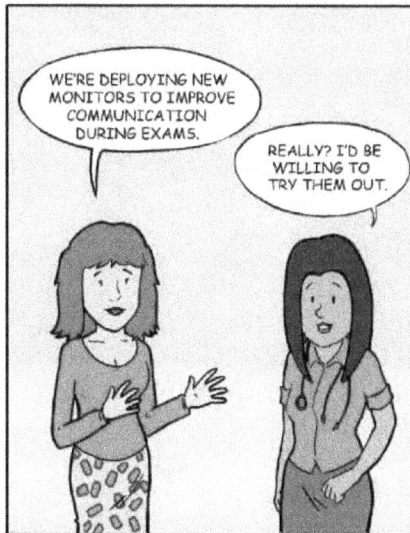

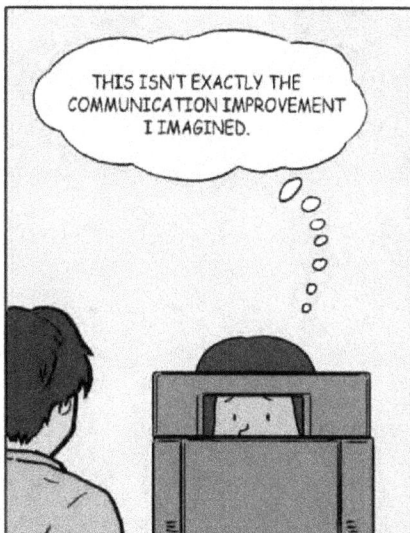

DOC-RELATED

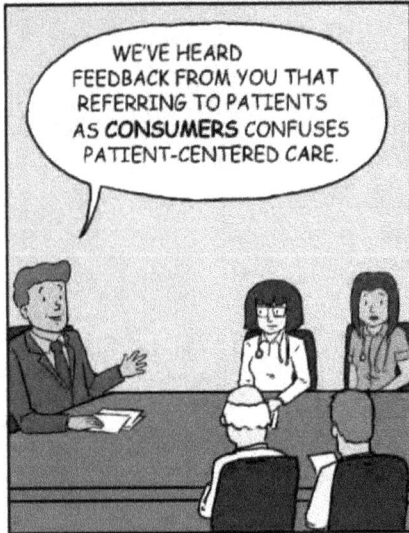

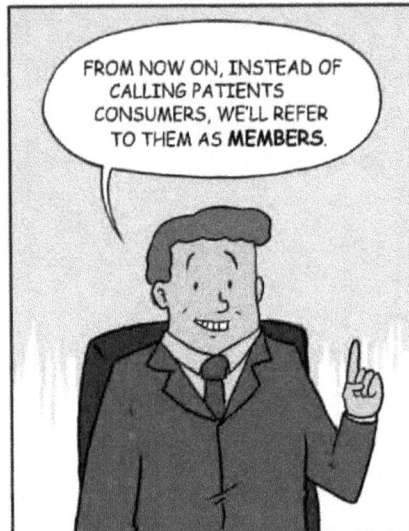

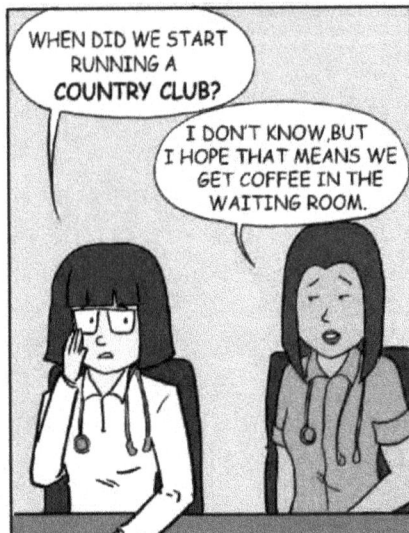

Dr. Peter Valenzuela

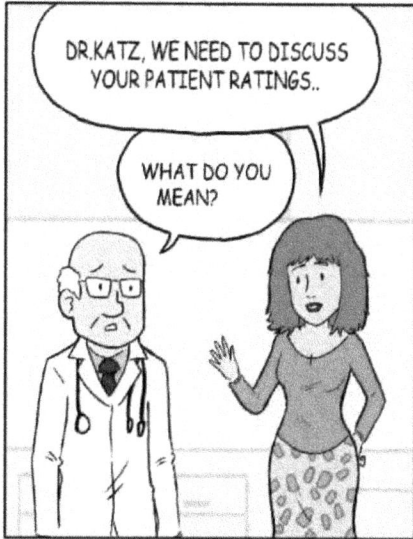

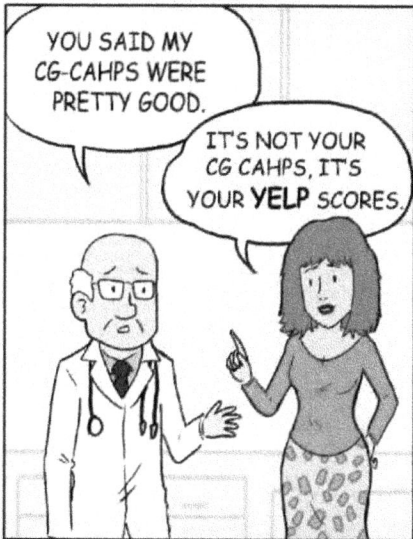

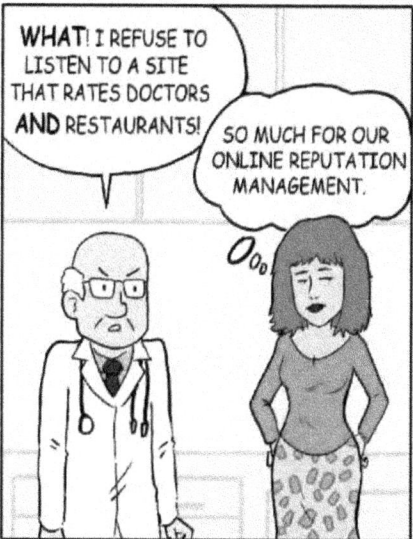

DOC RELATED

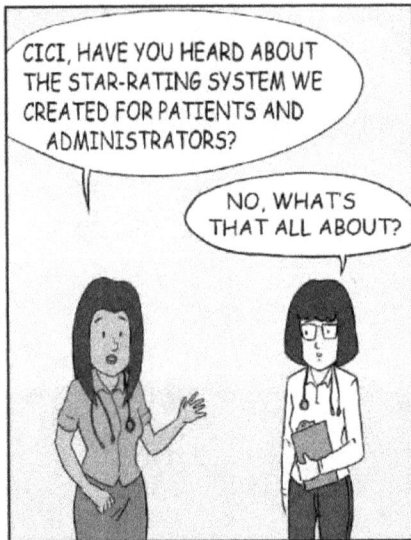

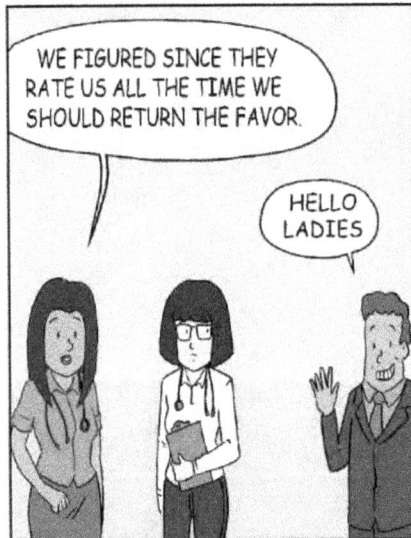

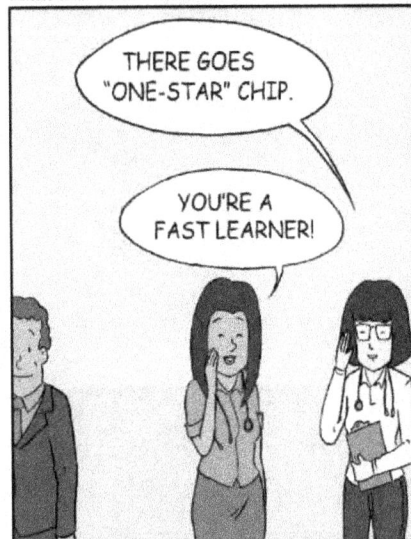

Dr. Peter Valenzuela

Chapter 3
Leadership & Communication: What Are You Saying?

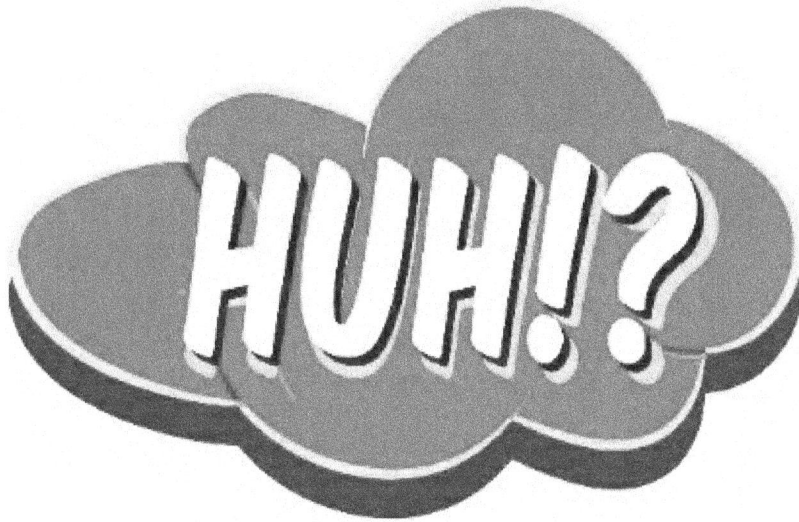

HUH!?

I had a boss who taught me relationships are all about trust and communication. But sometimes, what we say is not what the other person hears. This holds true for patients, too. I remember being a medical student working at the VA hospital in Dallas, listening to the surgery resident on our team talk with a patient about his anemia.

He said, "Sir, we need to find out where you're losing blood, so we're going to put a scope in your rectum to look around your colon. Then we're going to scope you through the mouth to look around your stomach. Do you have any questions?" I can still see the patient's eyes bulging and hear his voice trembling as he asked, "Are you going to wash the scope after you take it out of my rectum and put it in my mouth?" Our team tried its best not to laugh as the resident explained we would use two different scopes. Again, sometimes what we say is not what the other person hears.

Miscommunication doesn't just happen between doctors and patients, but with doctors and management as well. I've sat in meetings where executives used beautiful imagery and inspiring quotes to describe the current state of the organization. At times, they disconnected their statements from what staff and clinicians were experiencing on the frontline. Sometimes it felt like practicing physicians and administrators were speaking different languages. Unfortunately, this is not uncommon. In many organizations, trust is at an all-time low because of poor communication between administrators and physicians.

Recently, I came across a physician engagement study that investigated the differences between physicians and hospital administrators. First, analyses of language and context revealed conflicting connotations related to power dynamics. For example, "increasing transparency and communication" meant different things to different participants. Half of the administrators and physicians interpreted this to mean "getting *them* onboard" or "helping *them* understand" rather than building two-way dialogue to address issues. "Being present" also had different connotations. Half of the responders interpreted this to mean policing the other side's activities to make sure they are doing the work. The other half interpreted "being present" as caring about staff and being available to support the department.

Compared to physicians, administrators also had a much more positive perception of hospital systems and initiatives — which might explain why situations may seem better to administrators in meetings. This in no way means the administrators are incorrect. On paper, administrators may be accurately describing the performance of the organization based on its targets or dashboards. However, physicians measure performance as it pertains to patient care and day-to-day work. Below is a prime example of comments from study participants after implementing a centralized call center:

Administrator: "Now there's a centralized scheduling system. It's one number, one pool of people. If the call center gets 60,000 calls and you have two mistakes this week, well, they're human. That's not the worst of errors."

Physician: "Do they know us? Of course not. How could they know hundreds of physicians? They don't know whether we specialize in this or that, and sometimes people are scheduled completely wrong. If someone cancels, anybody with a random condition will take that spot even though it could be something completely idiotic for me to see."

At the core of this disconnect is understanding the challenges each faces. Physicians may believe they are being treated like assembly line workers making as many widgets — or in this case, seeing as many patients — as possible. They are not being asked about staffing or strategies to be successful. On the other side, administrators working in large organizations may believe that doctors are unaware of what it takes to keep the lights on operationally and financially.

This segues into the next big difference the research noted between physicians and administrators: problem-solving. Study findings show administrators addressed problems differently. They distilled information into multiple options over an extended period (weeks to months). I imagine that much of this is wanting to tackle the right problem in the right way instead of throwing additional staffing resources at it.

Physicians were more likely to distill information into one best course of action within minutes to days. This is a byproduct of medical training and the need to make quick decisions in diagnosis and treatments. The administrative mindset for deferred decision-making played a big role in physician frustration and poor engagement in this study. It was also challenging for administrators dealing with impatient physicians.

Why do these differences matter?

I've learned that organizations don't have values. Sure, they may have mission, vision, and value statements on their walls, but ultimately, organizations take on the values of their leaders. This establishes organizational culture. Ideally, leaders should protect others from stress and be cool under pressure. Some leaders are more likely to cause stress than to reduce it. This stress can lead to employee burnout. The problem is far more common than it should be, especially in the health care industry.

From a professional perspective, burnout can decrease quality of care and increase medical errors. Burnout also leads to higher physician turnover rates and less productivity. From a personal perspective, burnout leads to broken relationships with higher incidences of alcohol and substance abuse. Even more alarming is the rate of depression and suicide in physicians who are burned out.

Conservative figures estimate doctor burnout costs the U.S. health care system roughly $4.6 billion a year. Still, it only factors lost work hours and physician turnover. It doesn't factor in the cost of medical mistakes, less satisfied patients, or malpractice suits.

Dr. Tate Shanafelt's research on burnout and physician satisfaction highlights the role of leadership in health care. He's found that every 1-point increase in leadership score is associated with a 3.3% decrease in the likelihood of burnout and a 9.0% increase in clinician satisfaction. Essentially, 11% of the variation in burnout and 47% of the variation in satisfaction are connected to how well clinicians rated their leaders.

What Type of Leaders Should We Have?

Along with aligned communication and collaborative relationships with physicians, we need strong leaders who truly understand patient-centered care and can focus on clinical outcomes. It's not surprising to find that organizations led by physicians perform better. Hospital quality scores are approximately 25 percent higher in physician-run hospitals than in manager-run hospitals. The same is true in high-performing medical groups with physician-led governance structures. They do well because physicians maintain control over key decisions, particularly those affecting clinical care and day-to-day practice operations.

In addition, a Front Line of Healthcare Survey found that, at physician-led groups, physicians tend to be more satisfied with their employer. Approximately 80 percent feel inspired by the organization's mission, and 83 percent feel sufficiently engaged in decisions about strategic direction. This is understandable. Studies have linked people who are experts in their respective fields with better organizational performance in all arenas. I'm sure you can name at least a few athletes who became successful coaches after retirement. Being a basketball fan who loves the Spurs and Warriors, Doc Rivers and Steve Kerr come to mind. My tennis buddies often cite Ivan Lendl and Billie Jean King. For Chicago Bears fans, it's five letters — D-I-T-K-A. The list goes on and on.

When asked why physician-led organizations appear to do better, Dr. Toby Cosgrove, past CEO of Cleveland Clinic, responded without hesitation, "credibility... peer-to-peer credibility." When talented doctors lead organizations, they show that they have been in the physicians' shoes and have insights into their needs. I can't tell you how many times I've had a clinician tell me, "What do they (administration) know? They don't see patients." This is a big reason I continue to see patients as a physician leader today. I want to show my colleagues that I am in the trenches right there with them.

Early in the COVID-19 pandemic, there was a lot of fear in our medical group related to a novel virus few knew much about. Our clinicians were hesitant to work in the drive-thru respiratory clinic created to care for sick patients and perform COVID-19 screening. Understanding their concerns, I volunteered to be one of the first physicians to work in the clinic. My goal was to help streamline our process for those clinicians that followed me and to serve as a role model for the group. After all, you can't ask people to do something you're not willing to do yourself.

I must confess, after donning all my personal protective equipment (PPE), I was a little scared for my health. I was even more afraid that I might bring something home to my wife. After screening a few patients, I realized my gear would protect me, and I just needed to focus on doing what was best for the patient. Sharing my experience and vulnerability with the clinicians in our group went a long way in allaying fears and served as a lightning rod for others to volunteer.

Please know that some of the best bosses I've had in my 20-year career were NOT physicians. What they had in common was that they were all systems thinkers who could build strong relationships with health care professionals and influence outcomes. They were also curious and emotionally intelligent, with high integrity. For problem-solving or challenging situations, one of my bosses would always say, "Peter, don't tell me no, tell me how." She forced me to think differently, which often worked.

These characteristics are not always innate, so organizations should invest in leadership development as much as possible. Unfortunately, education and training are often the most underfunded and understaffed departments in many organizations. We view them as "nice to haves" instead of critical to success. Peter Baeklund coaches authentic leadership and peak performance. He's well known for the following quote:

> **CFO** asks CEO: What happens if we invest in developing our people and they leave?
> **CEO:** What happens if we don't, and they stay?

This quote especially applies to leadership development in health care. I often joke with clinicians that I went to back to school to get my MBA so I could translate what administrators say to terms more understandable for clinicians. It's surprising how helpful my MBA has been over the years — it's also been great for making comics. My MBA has taught me that terms like "right-sizing" and "optimize" really mean cutting staff and using the least amount of resources to do the most amount of work.

Although studies show that physician-led organizations fare better, finding well-rounded doctors with business acumen can be a challenge, especially when there are no formal training programs within the organization. It becomes more complicated when the physician leader is still medically practicing because clinical responsibilities take priority over meetings. Understanding this concept, some of the premiere health care organizations in the country have the best of both worlds via dyad leadership.

Dyad leadership is a partnership composed of an administrative leader and a physician leader. The key to dyadic success is to have clear lines of communication and roles that are not overlapping. Physician leaders handle quality, patient care standards, clinical pathways, and clinician performance. Administrators oversee revenue management, staff recruiting and training, performance reports, and support systems. Both partners handle innovation, strategic planning, and the overall performance of the department. Both partners have the authority to make critical changes when necessary. Although the Mayo Clinic established this structure over 100 years ago, it hasn't completely caught on across the U.S. Many organizations are still led by administrators with no clinical partners.

The Accountable Leader by Brian Dive stresses the importance of establishing and maintaining clear structures. The book identifies three concepts of successful corporations, including leadership, accountability, and organizational structure. Dyad leadership uses matrix reporting, where an employee works for a direct supervisor while also reporting to another leader in the organization. Most commonly, physicians report to a physician leader, and support staff report to the administrator.

A Word of Caution

When done well, matrix reporting structures can be great for organizations. However, some organizations can go overboard with reporting structures and org charts that may blur oversight and accountabilities. Often, the larger the organization, the more layers of administrative bureaucracy. At one point in my career, I had four leaders that I reported to at work while still reporting to my wife at home!

One of my favorite — although somewhat heretical books — is *First, Let's Fire All the Managers.* It points out that multiple layers of management can be detrimental to organizations because:

1.   As organizations grow, management overhead increases incrementally and may account for as much as 33 percent of payroll.

2.   Traditional hierarchies increase the risk of large, disastrous decisions because of the limited number of individuals who can challenge the decision. This is especially true when the "uncontestable" leader decides.

3.   Not uncommonly, plans created by those too far from the work are unsuccessful.

4.   Multiple layers of management translate to additional levels of approval and the inability to effect a change in a timely fashion.

Ways to Fix Leadership and Communication

Miscommunication between physicians and administrators leads to rumors and distrust. When Nancy Steiger was CEO of PeaceHealth's Northwest Network, she focused on improving communication and dispelling myths. She held regular in-person town hall meetings for all the staff. She also set up CEO-physician forums and dedicated a section of the forum to "Rumors and True-mors." It provided the doctors an opportunity to ask timely questions about the direction of the organization and voice any concerns they may have. Nancy had a background as an oncology nurse, and she had a way of communicating with physicians that exuded trust.

Along with opening lines of communication, we should allow physicians and administrators to walk in each other's shoes. In the *Art of Innovation*, Tom Kelley states, "If you're not in the jungle, you're not going to know the tiger." To know the stressors others face, you need to expose yourself to their environment. Exposing administrators to the realities of patient care — via shadowing physicians or attending team huddles in care units or clinics — can provide them a deeper understanding of these decisions on patients, clinicians, and the clinical workplace. Shadowing has the potential to provide administrators with more insight in a day than they could learn in multiple meetings over months.

On the other side, physicians should gain an understanding about leadership and the red tape administrators must deal with running the business. Although some physicians have innate leadership abilities, all can benefit from formal development. One of the best ways to do this is to earn an MBA or master's in health care administration (MHA), but that is easier said than done for practicing physicians. Earning a master's degree is time-consuming and expensive.

Another option is to enroll in employer-sponsored training programs. Physicians can also seek coaching or mentoring within their organization or through their professional societies.

Perhaps an easier approach is to take part in committees to better understand the inner workings of the organization. Just like for administrators shadowing physicians, physicians can shadow administrators to learn more about their day.

Establishing dyads can also bridge the leadership gap, so everyone is rowing in the same direction. In addition, health care needs to learn how to be organizationally nimble to implement change. Too many layers of approval will hinder innovation and continue to frustrate clinicians. It is possible to be a big company and still be organizationally nimble.

Illinois Tool Works (ITW) is a $14 billion company that manufactures a wide range of products, including industrial packaging and food equipment. To continue its success, ITW thinks small. Once a business unit reaches $200 million in revenue, they divide the unit into two $100 million units. The company would rather have ten independently run, innovative $100 million units than a single monolithic $1 billion unit.

To enhance communication and build trust, we need to incorporate the physician's voice in management conversations. It's vital to have the right people in leadership roles who share the same perceptions and cultures as those on the frontlines. These leaders will help elevate priorities and patient outcomes. To nurture physician and clinician leadership, organizations need to invest in leadership development programs. Finally, we need to regularly assess leaders by those they lead.

Although this seems like a straightforward decision, organizations measure most health care leaders by how they perform on targets and scorecards. But it's important for leaders to be measured by how they interact with and treat others in the department. Essentially, we need to be the leaders we wish to see. After all when it boils down to it, "It's all about trust and communication."

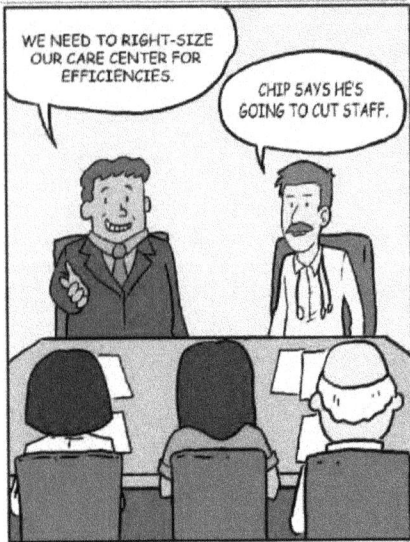

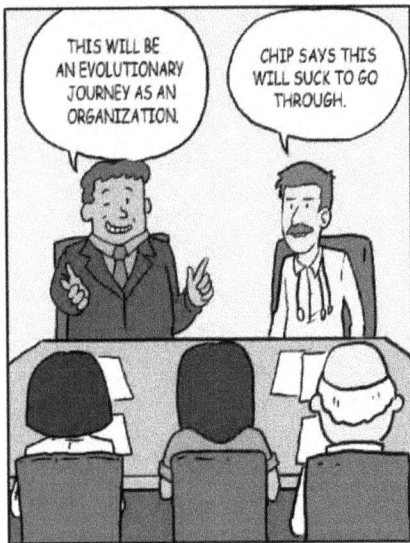

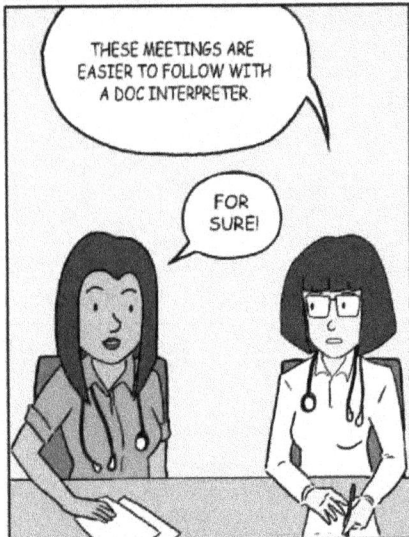

Dr. Peter Valenzuela

DOC ⬤RELATED

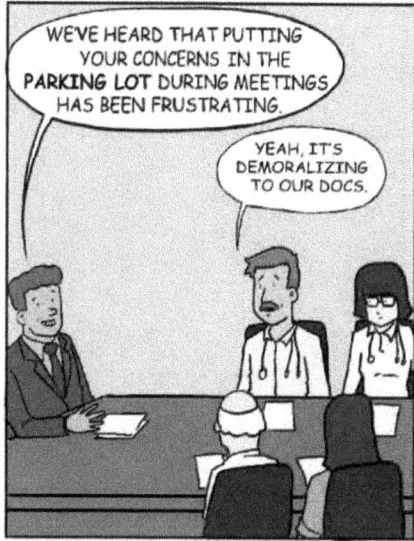

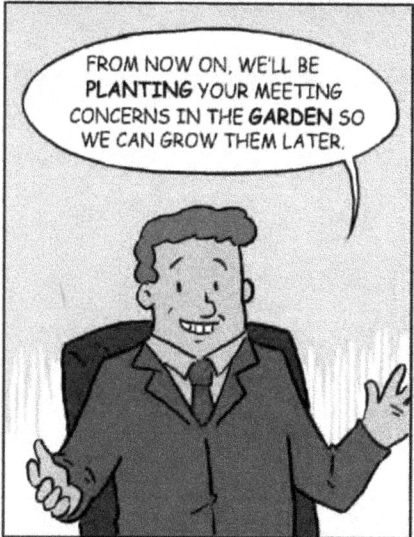

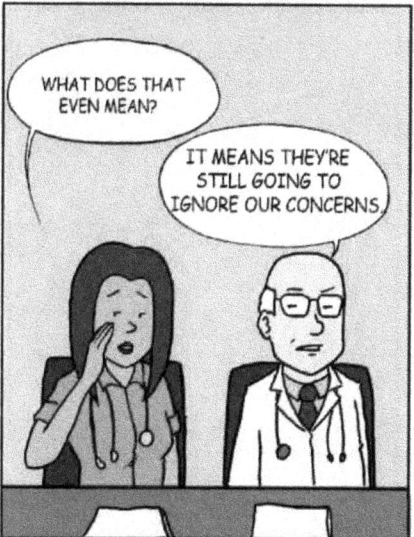

Dr .Peter Valenzuela

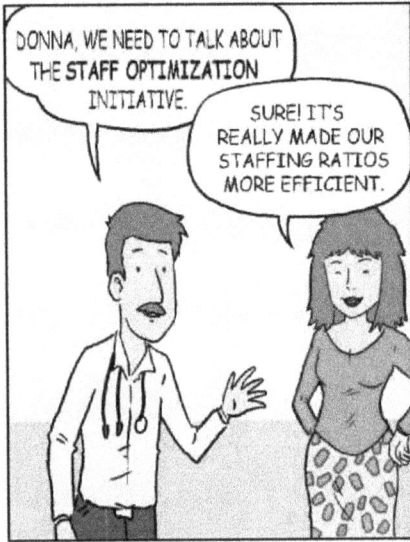

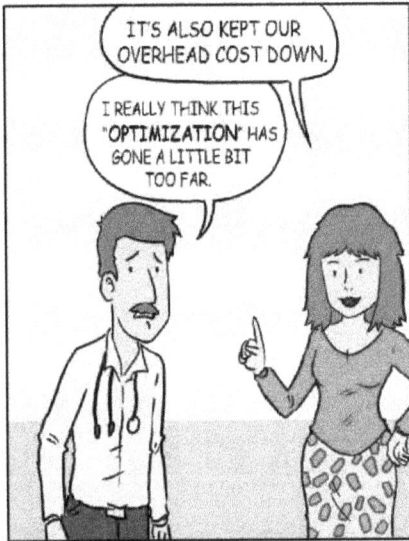

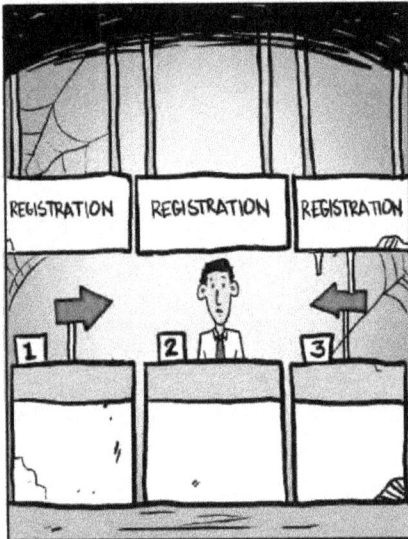

Dr. Peter Valenzuela

DOC RELATED

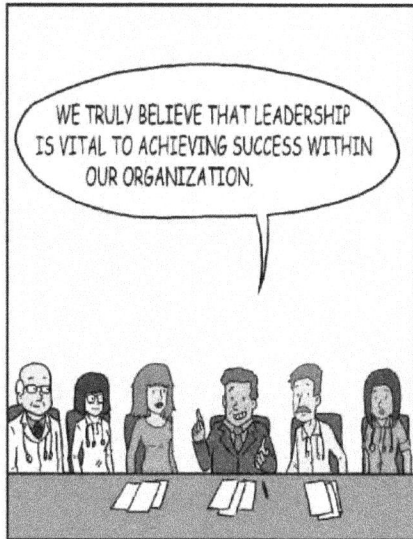

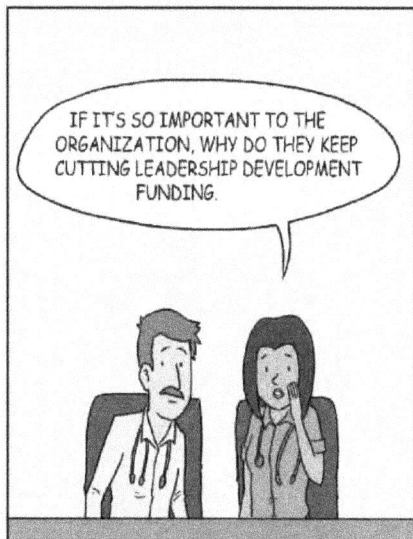

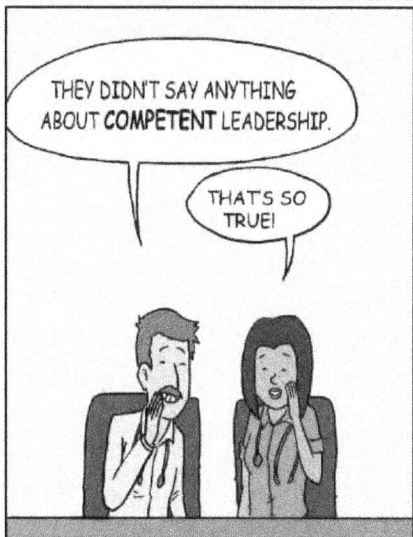

Dr. Peter Valenzuela

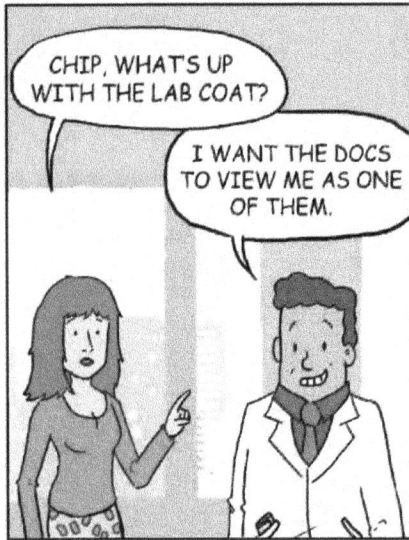

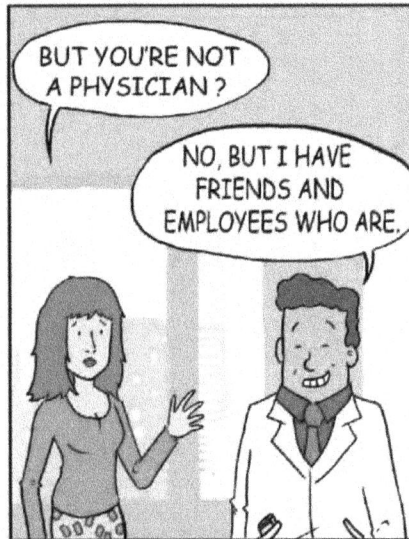

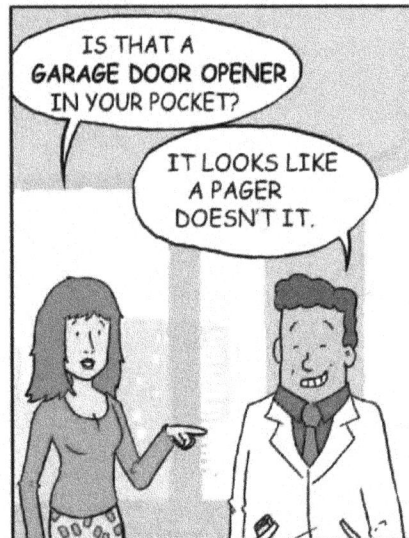

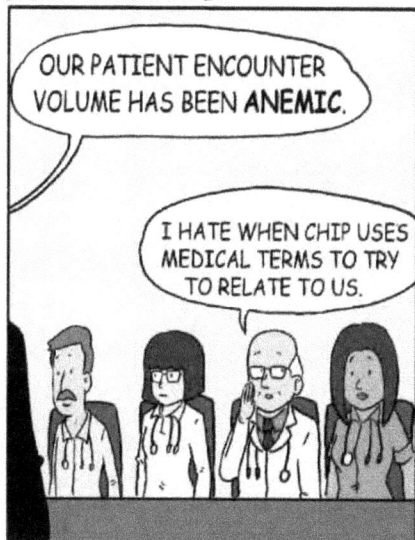

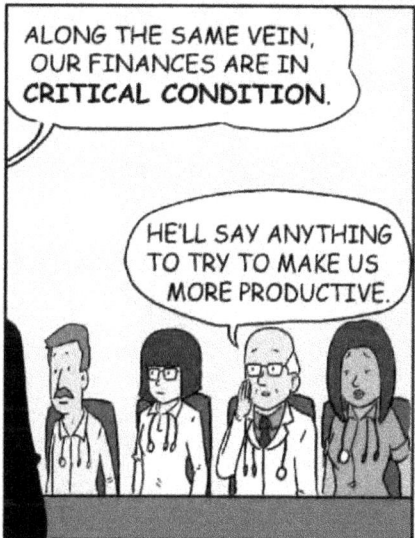

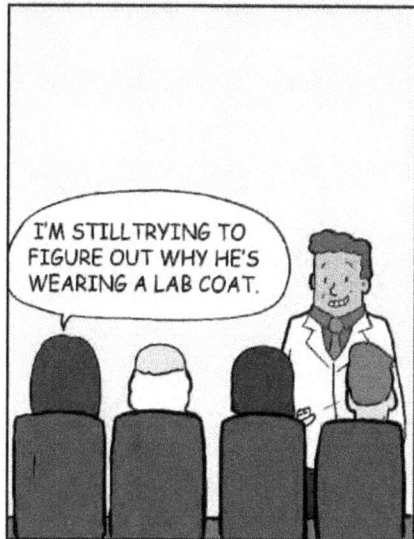

Dr. Peter Valenzuela

DOC RELATED

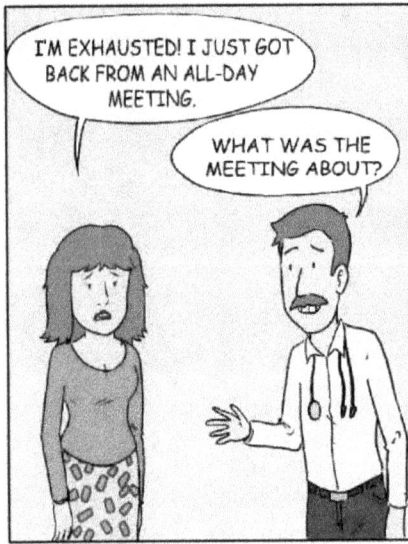

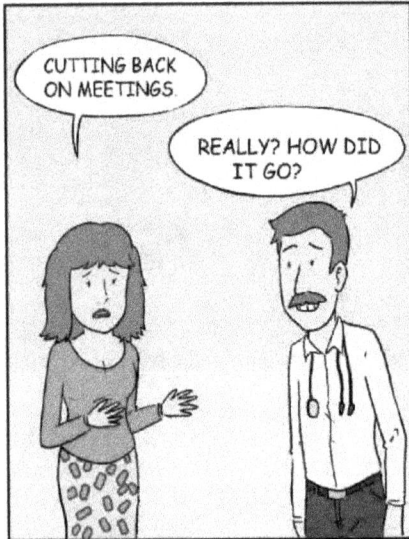

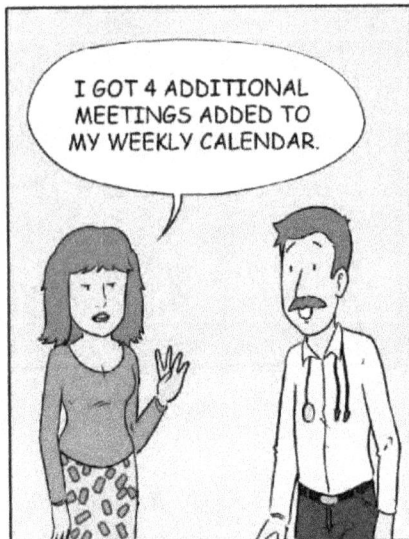

Dr. Peter Valenzuela

DOC RELATED

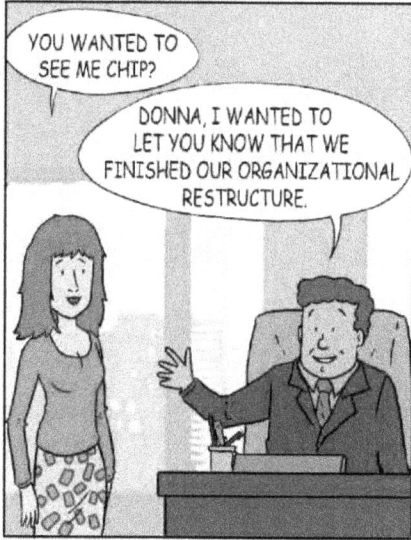

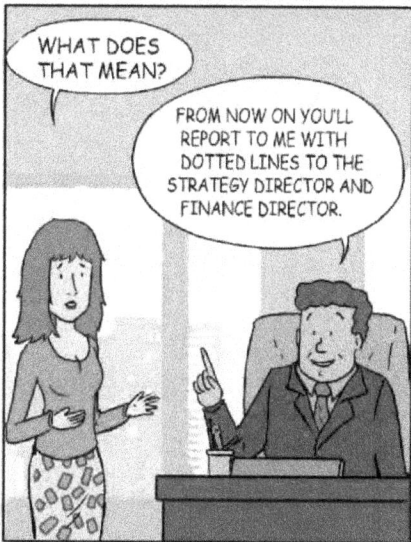

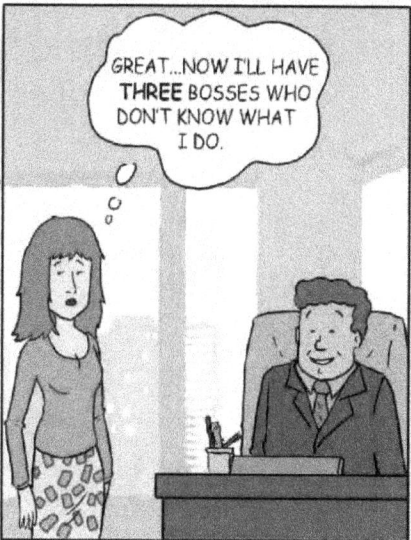

Dr. Peter Valenzuela

DOC RELATED

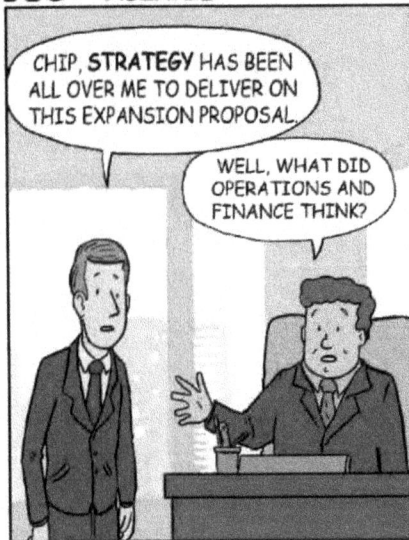

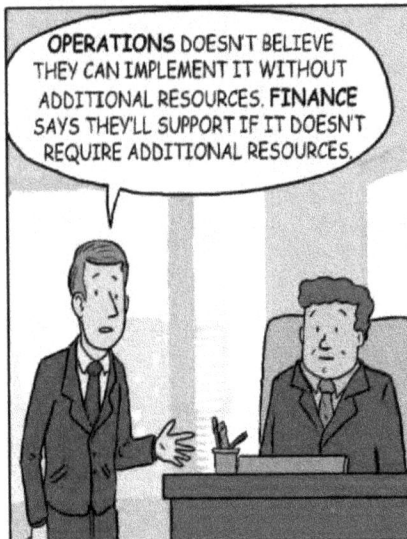

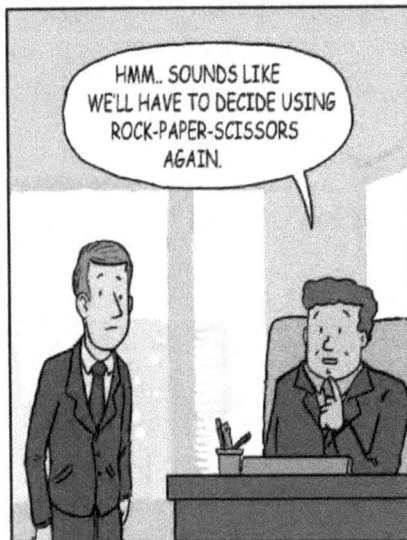

Dr. Peter Valenzuela

DOC ◄■► RELATED

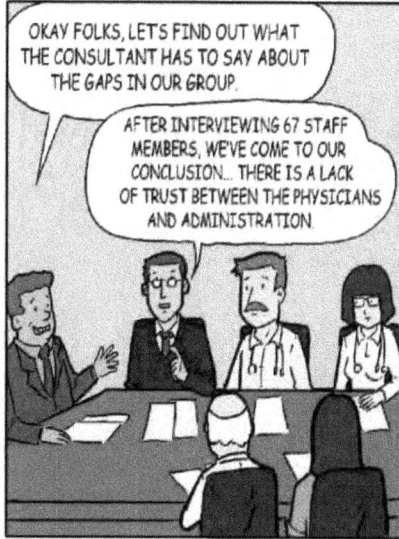

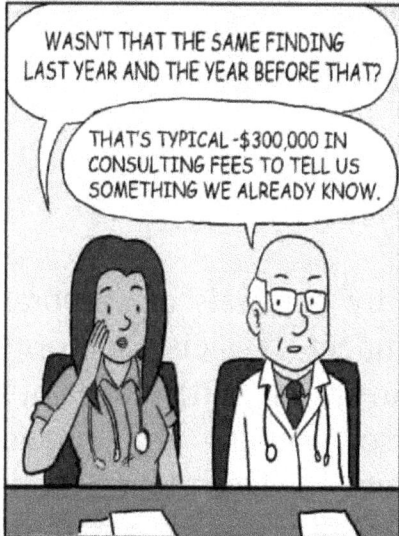

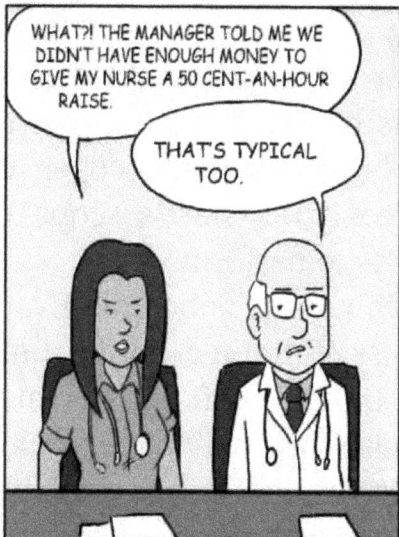

Dr. Peter Valenzuela

Chapter 4
Staff & Resources: Do You Have What You Need?

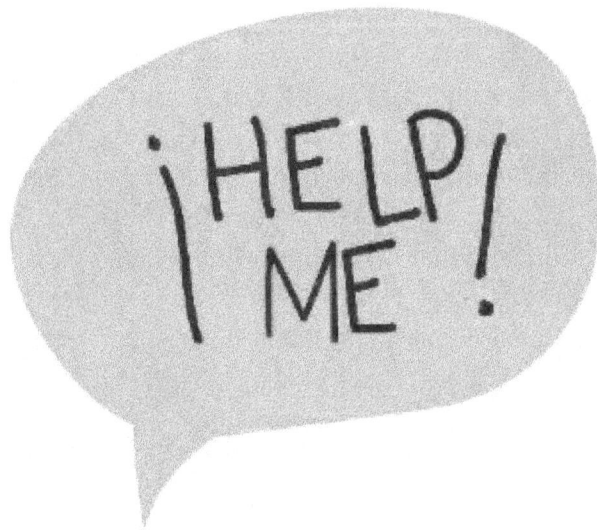

Today, with more physicians being employed by hospitals or corporate entities, decisions related to staffing are no longer under physician authority. Although some organizations include physicians in hiring staff, most must work with what they provide. Because personnel are the biggest organizational expense, hiring staff is heavily monitored. Departments must justify the need to bring on more staff. As a result, clinics end up competing for staff support when funds are tight.

If the care center can hire staff, it may not be the type needed to complete the work. For example, medical assistants have different scopes of licensure than licensed vocational nurses, who have different scopes of licensure than registered nurses. Whatever is beyond the staff's scope of licensure becomes the responsibility of the physicians to perform.

Besides the type of support provided, staff training and onboarding vary from one department to another. Often, this process is limited due to time constraints or lack of training personnel. Poorly trained staff also creates more work for those that are trained correctly because they may have to pick up the slack, which can also lead to turnover. This results in the remaining staff being forced to take on additional coverage responsibilities, which puts them at risk of burnout. It's no wonder that vacancy rates for nurses run at 17%.

Because many large employers have policies that favor the employee on leave—and because they cannot fill a position for a person on leave of absence — they're forced to use float pools to help those departments needing support. Unfortunately, it's impossible to train float staff to adequately cover every specialty. Primary care clinics have different needs from medical specialty clinics and surgical specialty clinics. Besides differences in specialty needs, there are differences in physician styles and preferences. This again results in physicians providing services that may be better handled by clinical staff.

Another strategy used to save on cost is to centralize support. On the plus side, centralization can ease work that gets pushed to physicians and staff. However, organizations need to be cautious in deciding what should be centralized. In addition, removing a 1.0 full-time equivalent (FTE) staff person from the care center may result in only 50-75% of centralized support. This leaves the rest of the work being previously done by the person removed for others to perform at the care center.

As I write this book, we continue to deal with COVID. Organizations have shifted from in-person visits to virtual encounters. The biggest reason for the transition is the safety of patients and staff. Although they've been around for a while, we made virtual visits more workable because the government loosened privacy restrictions and payers agreed to pay for them at the same rate as in-person visits.

Many in health care hope this will be our new future and that it will cut back on the need for staff. Virtual care is convenient for some populations with a level of technological savvy who have internet or mobile access. However, older and underserved populations struggle to navigate video visits and require more staff time to train the patient and prepare for a visit.

Ways to Fix Staffing and Operations

An ideal practice will have the right people performing the right jobs. Vital to having the right people is properly training them to do the work. For example, pharmacists and RNs should fill prescriptions and triage patients. Social workers and care managers should assist patients in getting what they need at home and ensuring they follow up for care. Medical assistants and front desk staff should properly handle messages and respond to patients when possible. The cost savings from more productive clinicians will more than offset the additional staff investment.

According to the Medical Group Management Association (MGMA), better performing practices reported almost 9% greater medical total operating cost per full-time-equivalent (FTE) physician than their peers. These groups also had substantially greater total medical revenue per FTE physician, showing that investments in staff, facilities, and operations pay off in the bottom line.

Centralization can help supplement work for staff and physicians on the frontline. However, it should not be used in place of providing essential staff to care for patients. Strategic decisions for moving services to central offices — or remotely — should prioritize the effect on the patient, the physician, and the staff. Otherwise, short-term cost savings may cause long-term absenteeism and turnover. It will also impact the ability for patients to receive timely care.

If necessary, floating staff from one care center to another should be done in a coordinated fashion. Sutter Gould Medical Group is recognized as one of the best medical groups in the country by the American Medical Group Association (AMGA). They look at schedules weeks in advance. When they see a department that will have physicians out of the office for an extended period, they assure the office has adequate coverage support. Next, they approach support staff and ask if they will work in another care center. If the staff agrees, they will send them to that care center to be trained prior to actually working their shifts. Staff members appreciate getting paid to learn and having variety in their work. Doctors are grateful to have trained coverage when their regular staff are out.

To have well-designed systems, we need to apply Lean strategies based on the Toyota Production System (TPS). One Lean technique used to help design large-scale improvements is catchball. In catchball, the person starting a project describes the problem, objective, and any other ideas to other stakeholders for feedback and support. This helps to create bi-directional feedback and solve problems at the point of care.

Another Lean strategy is the use of variation reduction to implement care standards. This is critical to improving quality and decreasing waste. For example, care centers should agree on rooming standards for staff that will help gain efficiencies and allow anyone filling in to be quickly trained. Supply rooms should undergo 5S. This is a Lean term that stands for Sort, Set in Order, Shine, Standardize, and Sustain. It's used to organize, clean, develop, and sustain a productive work environment. Using 5S eases frustrations of not being able to find equipment and supplies at the time of care. When done well — and including those on the frontlines — implementing Lean techniques can identify efficiencies and streamline patient throughput. Lean will also decrease errors and improve patient care.

Besides Lean, we need to apply design thinking to transform the clinician experience of providing care. Both Lean and design thinking rely on bringing clinical team members together to improve care processes. Lean has been in the healthcare industry for decades but has taken a while to find success. Design thinking has only recently been introduced to health care but is gaining traction. The ideology behind design thinking is that a hands-on, user-centric approach to problem-solving can lead to innovation. Innovation can lead to differentiation and a competitive advantage. Design thinking employs empathy to explore how users — in our case, physicians, clinicians, and staff — do their work, think, and feel about their environment. Like Lean, design thinking follows a process of first understanding the problem, exploring potential solutions, and finally materializing the best option. Where Lean targets efficiencies in throughput, design-thinking targets process transformations with a focus on how people feel.

With appropriate staffing and techniques that engage all stakeholders, we can create a supportive work community where people figure out how to work out problems and trust each other. This will provide an environment where physicians and staff have everything they need to be successful.

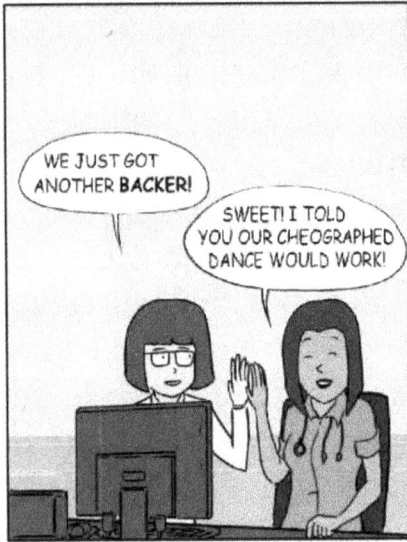

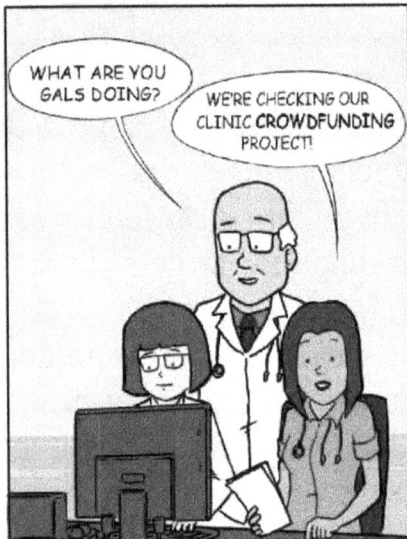

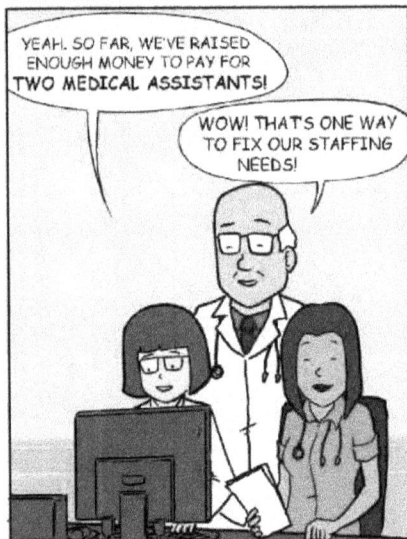

Dr. Peter Valenzuela

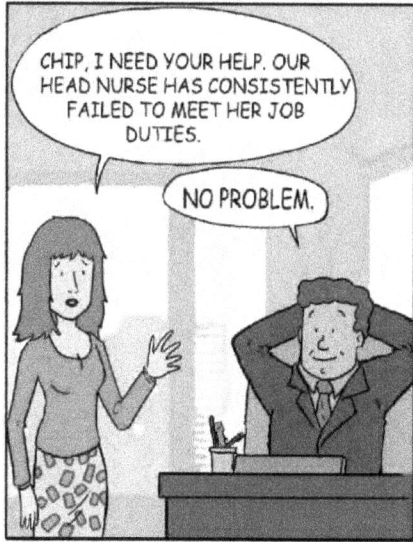

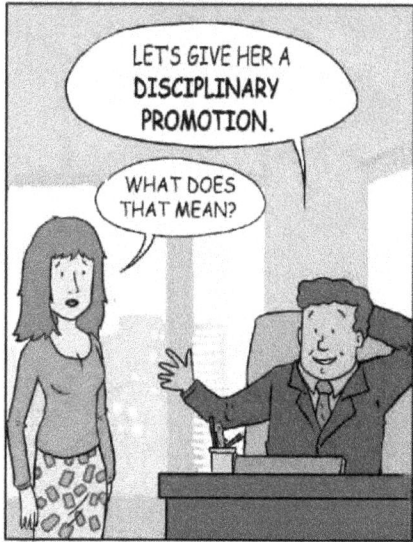

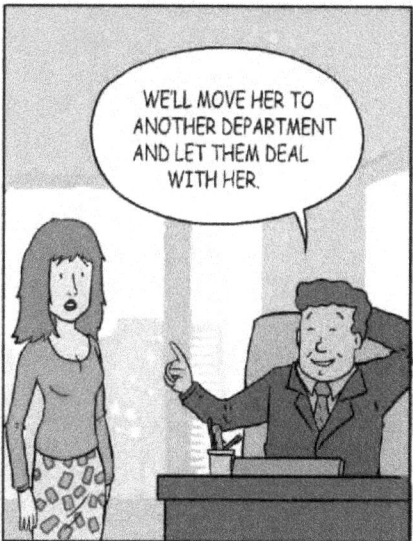

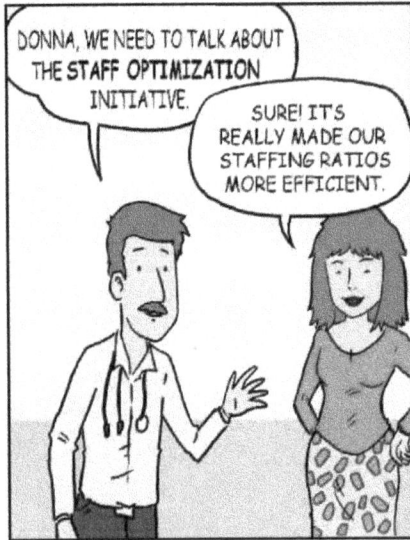

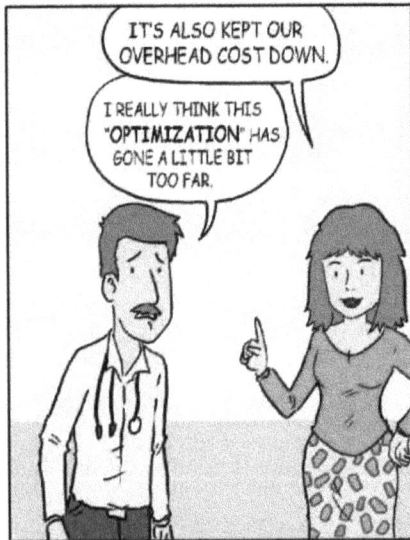

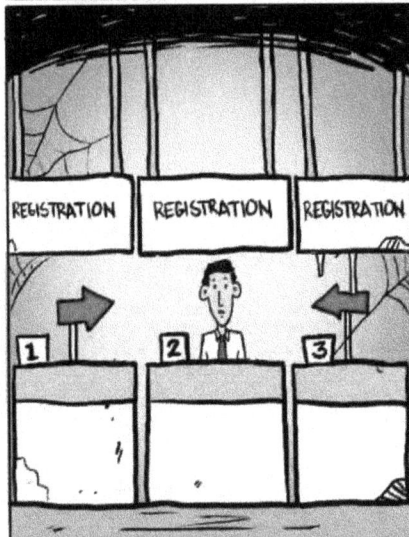

Dr. Peter Valenzuela

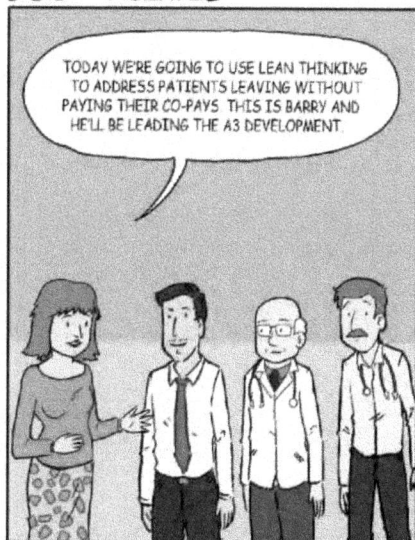

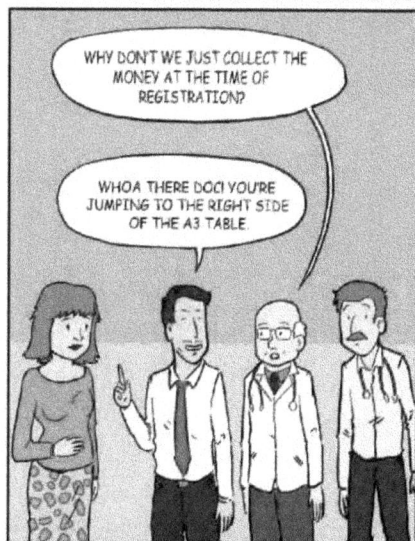

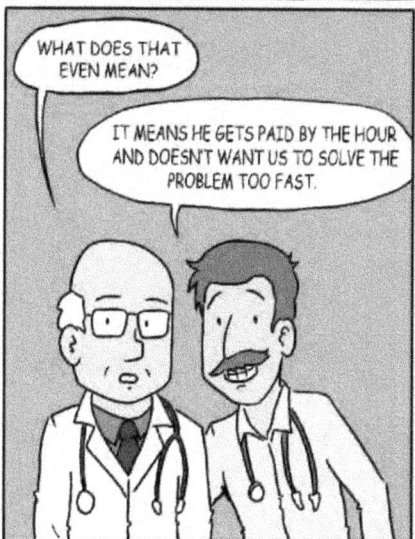

Dr. Peter Valenzuela

Part 2:
Payment

Chapter 5
Health Insurance: Will This Be Covered?

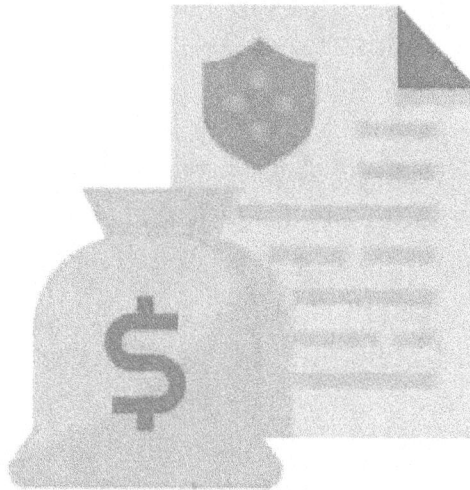

Here's a little secret: Most docs don't know what insurance will cover when they see a patient. For business-savvy physicians out there, this may sound like blasphemy. However, employed physicians now exceed those that own their practice. Many chose employed models because they didn't want to deal with insurance hassles. With patients inquiring more about the cost of services, along with pre-authorization requirements and referral restrictions, insurance has created a new form of frustration for physicians and clinicians. These frustrations include time-consuming activities like excess paperwork and unnecessary questions.

To understand this frustration, we must understand the complexities of health insurance. There are over 900 health insurance companies offering medical coverage in the U.S. Government-run health coverage—including Medicare, Medicaid, and Tricare—is the biggest provider of insurance in the U.S., caring for approximately 43% of the population.

The five largest private companies include Anthem, UnitedHealthcare, Humana, Health Care Service Corporation (HCSC), and CVS Health Corp., control over 44% of the market. Besides the number of insurance providers, there are multiple types of plans. Each plan has its own coverage, premium, deductible, copay, and co-insurance amounts. I've been teaching practice management to physicians for the last 15 years, and they still struggle to distinguish between the different types of insurance, the coverages they provide, and the costs and responsibilities associated.

Insurance Plans

Here is a list of the most common insurance plans, a brief description of these plans, and a few pain points for docs:

- Health maintenance organizations (HMOs)
- Preferred provider organizations (PPOs)
- Exclusive provider organizations (EPOs)
- Point-of-service (POS) plans
- High-deductible health plans (HDHPs)

An HMO delivers all health services through a network of healthcare providers and facilities for a monthly fee. Premiums are lower because of additional restrictions to HMO members. In this model, a primary care doctor is assigned to manage the care of the patient and is paid a dollar amount per member per month, regardless of whether the patient comes into the office.

Although this sounds great conceptually, it may translate to lots of virtual care via online messages, telephone encounters, and video visits for clinicians. These types of interactions can be helpful for the patient experience but can negatively affect physician wellness since completion of this work often occurs after hours. HMO savings also occur in part because of the layers of approval required to order high-cost procedures and ancillaries. In addition, making referrals can be a challenge because of limitations in-network specialists and the need to get pre-authorizations by the insurance company.

Unlike an HMO, patients have more freedom to choose their physicians in a PPO, and they don't need a referral to see specialists. If patients use out-of-network physicians, they may have to pay that physician directly and then file a claim to get the PPO plan to pay them back. Because patients are not always the most knowledgeable about their conditions, they may request unnecessary procedures or services they believe they need.

This is compounded by the fact that providers caring for patients in PPO models are paid based on procedures and services, so they may be more motivated to increase services. Both patients and providers can make health care costs higher in PPOs when not closely monitored.

Much like a PPO, an EPO offers patients a moderate amount of freedom to choose their physicians. They also don't need a referral from a primary care doctor to see a specialist. However, there is zero coverage for out-of-network providers other than in an emergency. In both the PPO and EPO plan, doctors are not paid unless the patient is seen.

A POS plan blends aspects of an HMO with a PPO. Patients have more freedom to choose their physicians like a PPO, but the primary care physician coordinates care and referrals to specialists like an HMO. Like PPOs, patients can also see out-of-network doctors but will be required to pay more.

The plan that is the source of so many patient questions and physician frustrations is the HDHP. The most common questions asked by patients revolve around costs for services or procedures, which can vary from one facility to another. Often, physicians lack access to this information, requiring them or their staff to spend additional time calling around for the patient.

An HDHP can be part of an HMO, PPO, EPO, or POS (Are you still with me?) HDHPs have lower monthly premiums but higher co-insurance, out-of-pocket costs, and deductibles (cost averages are approximately $1,400 for individual plans and $2,800 for a family). On the plus side, patients can offset their HDHPs by contributing to health savings accounts (HSA), which allows patients to pay for certain medical expenses with money free from federal taxes. On the downside, only about half of the employers and half of the employees contribute to HSAs.

The key concept behind HDHPs is to shift out-of-pocket expenses from insurers and employers to individuals assuming they will be more discriminant in their insurance products and engage in a higher degree of price shopping. In other words, HDHPs should reward "consumer-driven" healthcare. As previously mentioned, many patients lack sufficient knowledge and time to make informed choices. In fact, people with HDHPs are far more likely than those with traditional health plans to forgo or delay medical care or to be in a household that is having difficulty paying medical bills.

Along with the plans listed above, states have their own marketplace with tiered plans organized by level of benefits such as bronze, silver, gold, and platinum. Bronze plans have the least coverage and are the least expensive, while platinum plans have the most coverage and are the most expensive. The deductibles vary according to the plan. The least expensive plan (bronze) carries the highest deductible.

With all the insurance types—and plan choices within those types—it is difficult for the patient to keep it all straight, let alone a physician. Physicians and their staff spend countless hours dealing with insurance plans for patient services, authorizations, referrals, medications, and medical supplies. The hassles of dealing with them can be overwhelming. Each plan has its own preferences on how they wish to receive information, review documentation, and communicate expectations with providers.

Ways to Fix Insurance Challenges

We need to eliminate "the hassle factor" for physicians and health care providers. Hassle factors refer to the increasingly intrusive and often irrational administrative, regulatory review, and paperwork burdens being placed on patients and physicians by the government programs and other insurers. The most basic step is to take the hassles out of the hands of the physicians by dedicating financial counselors and navigators to guide patients through the health care coverage waters. Having clinicians discuss extra topics they may not clearly understand is not in the best interest of the patient or the clinician.

An intermediate step is to develop interoperability standards requiring better integration between insurance plans and EHRs. Almost all EHRs currently list the name of the insurance provider but cannot provide specific detail on the plan and tier. Currently, physicians can identify whether a patient is on a Blue Cross plan — they may even be able to distinguish it as a PPO — but likely cannot tell whether it is a bronze tier or high-deductible plan. Stronger interoperability would allow all members of the care team to provide patients with point-of-care information related to coverage and co-pays and costs for services and medications based on their specific insurance plan.

The third and most advanced step is to change the way we receive payments. One way to do this is to pay physicians ahead of time. Advanced payments have been referred to as subscription models and prospective payments. They operate like a Medicare Advantage model with an annual budget per patient that pays the doctor a set amount monthly to provide care. This model would provide reliable funding through prospective payments for clinicians and health care organizations. It also allows organizations to invest in digital frontdoors like virtual visits and advanced practice providers to make sure patients have access to care.

Another way to change how we receive payments is to move towards a single-payer system like other developed countries, including England, France, Germany, and Spain. A single-payer system would unburden physicians from all the rules of complex risk models and administrative bureaucracy. A recent poll showed most health care professionals in the U.S. support a single-payer system. Besides being favored by health care professionals, multiple analyses show that a single-payer system would reduce health expenditures while providing high-quality insurance to *all* U.S. residents. The savings would mostly come from simplified billing and negotiated drug price reductions.

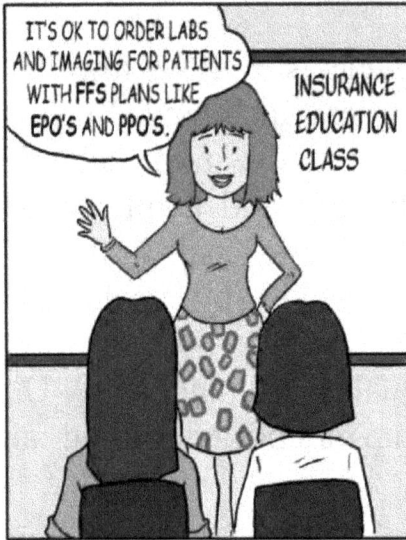

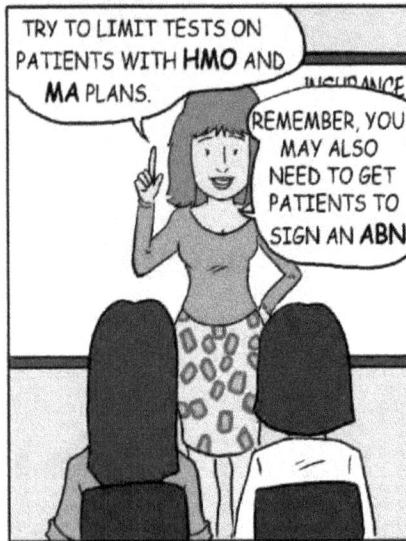

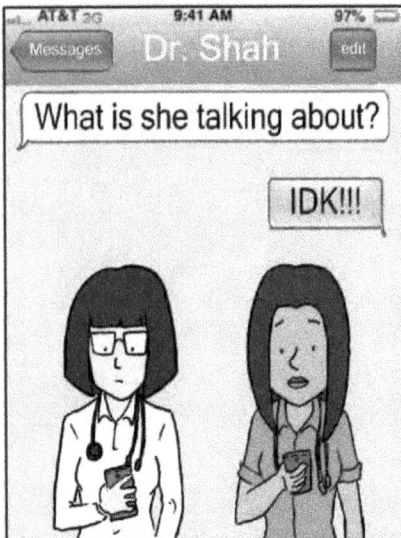

Dr. Peter Valenzuela

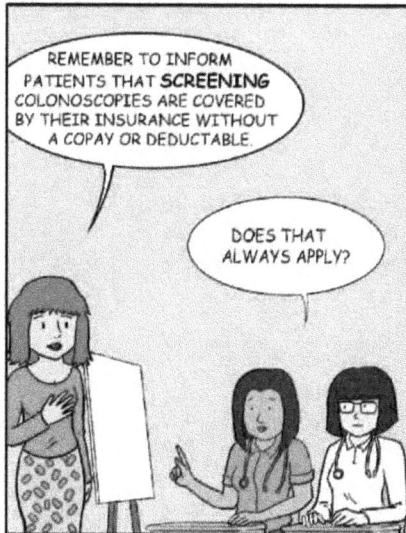

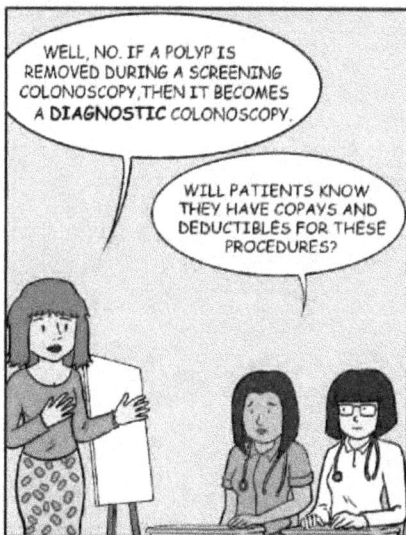

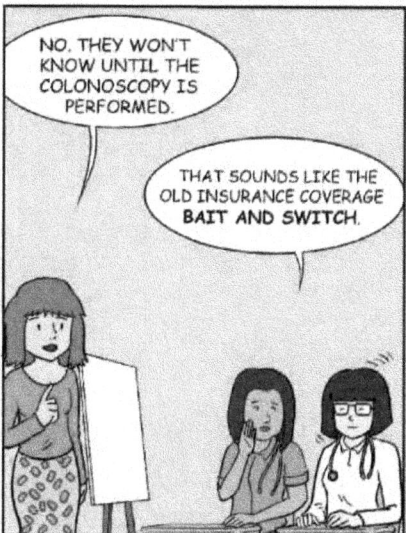

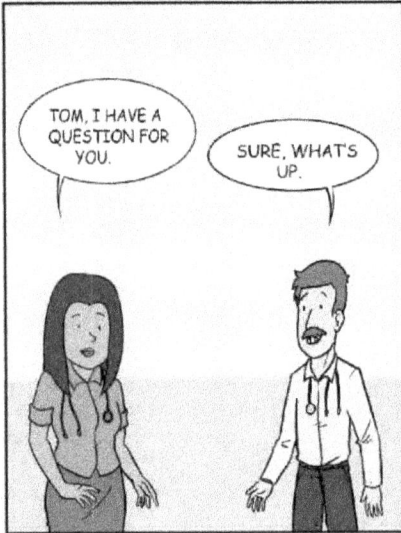

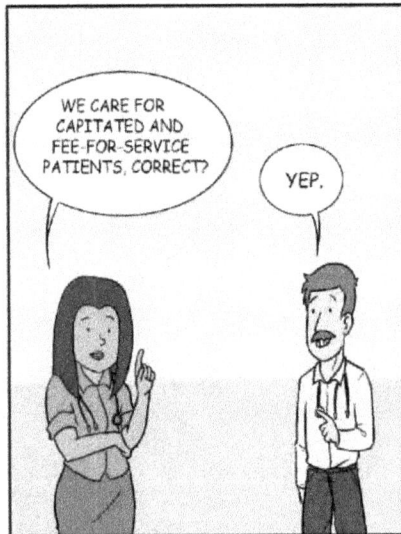

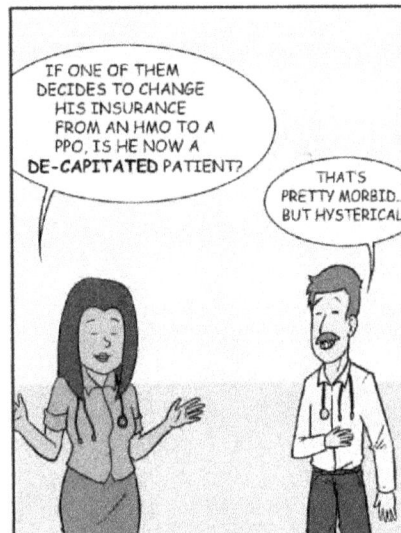

Chapter 6
Prior Authorization: You Need to Ask Me First

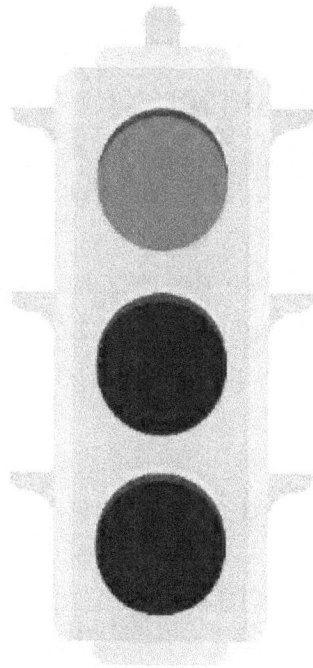

Dr. Glaucomflecken is an ophthalmologist and comedian with over 160,000 followers on Twitter. Like other physicians who satirize health care, he uses a pseudonym because, according to his site, "I can't quit my day job just yet, so I'm trying to protect myself from getting fired and my family from would-be assassins." One of his posts is a video re-enactment of a phone call with his insurance plan after suffering an acute cardiac arrest . It highlights both network coverage (making sure physicians providing services are contracted with the insurer) and seeking prior authorization for services:

> **Insurance Rep:** Good morning sir, how may I help you today?
> **Patient:** Hi, you guys are refusing to pay the bills for my emergency hospitalization because my doctor was out-of network.
> **Insurance Rep:** Yes, sir, that's correct.
> **Patient:** But the hospital I was taken to by ambulance was in -

network

Insurance Rep: Oh yes, sir, that's correct.

Patient: But the doctors that work inside the hospital were out of-network?

Insurance Rep: Some of them are in-network, but not yours.

Patient: How do you decide which doctors are in-network?

Insurance Rep: Well, they sign a contract allowing us to not pay them very much money.

Patient: But... not all doctors sign the contract?

Insurance Rep: Correct, like your doctors, sir.

Patient: But I didn't choose my doctors. I had a cardiac arrest and woke up in the ICU three days later.

Insurance Rep: Well, we do recommend patients (or their doctor's office) call us prior to using any medical services. There's a toll-free number on the back of your insurance card.

Although meant to be satirical, these cases occur frequently. So much so that obstetric patients are advised to make sure the hospital where they plan to give birth, along with the anesthesiologist providing the epidural, and the neonatal intensive care unit that may need to care for the baby, are all pre-approved by their insurance network before being admitted.

A prior authorization — or pre-auth — is a utilization management practice that health insurance companies require for certain procedures, tests, and medications prescribed by health care professionals. It assesses the medical necessity and cost-of-care ramifications of a service before it can be allowed. Insurance companies claim the purpose of pre-auths is to optimize patient outcomes by ensuring that they receive the most appropriate care while reducing waste and errors.

Before the 1980s, no one ever questioned how physicians cared for their patients. With the onset of managed care, they now call almost everything into question. This is especially true for high-ticket procedures and medications like surgeries that can safely occur in the outpatient setting, MRIs, durable medical equipment (DME), and specialty drugs.

Physicians don't just dislike pre-auths because they limit clinical autonomy, but they also consume lots of time and can be ridiculous, as Dr. Glaucomflecken points out. For example, when a physician prescribes gabapentin — a drug commonly used for certain types of nerve pain — the staff may spend 10-30 minutes completing pre-auth forms for this medication when a patient can get it online at GoodRx for less than $6.

Another example is requesting a pre-auth for a glucometer machine so a diabetic can check their sugars at home. Without checking blood sugars, the patient risks hospitalization for complications from their disease, which can lead to higher health care costs. The list goes on and on, so much so that the American Medical Association has a website dedicated to patient and physician stories dealing with pre-auths .

To understand the pain of pre-auths, you must know just how much information is requested, often in handwritten form. Below is a typical pre-auth form:

- Patient's name, gender, date of birth, address, health insurance identification number, and other contact information
- Identifying information for the referring provider (usually PCP) and servicing provider (treating physician). This can include contextual information, such as:
  o Referring provider information, including the name, national provider identifier (NPI).
  o Servicing provider information, including name and NPI number.
  o Clinical information specific to the treatment requested that the payer can use to establish medical necessity, such as: service type requiring authorization. This could include categories like ambulatory, acute, home health, dental, outpatient therapy, or durable medical equipment.
  o Service start date

- CPT and ICD codes

Not only is completing the form time-consuming, but the whole pre-auth process is challenging. First, the onus is on the health care provider to check a health plan's policy rules or formulary to determine if they require a prior authorization.

Second, clinical and healthcare billing systems are rarely integrated, so staff often must manually review prior authorization rules for the patient's specific insurance plan. These pre-auth rules tend to be found in archaic paper documentation or payer web portals. Not only that, but the payer rules aren't standardized and differ from health plan to health plan. The rules also change so frequently that a physician's staff may reference rules out of date. Finally, the responsibility falls on the physician's office to continue to follow up with the insurance company until there's a resolution of the pre-auth request.

A prior authorization can take anywhere from one day to several months to process. All the hoops to jump through leaves room for error. It's no wonder that 70% of payers say that they deny requests because what we sent over contradicts their guidelines.   I could write an entire chapter dedicated to prior auth denials. Denials are even more cumbersome and time-consuming.

Consider being a physician dealing with pre-auth requests multiple times a day for imaging, labs, medications, equipment, and procedures you believe are medically necessary. Now imagine trying to justify your reasoning to non-physicians following algorithms that don't always fit the patient. On the rare occasions they elevate a request to a physician within the insurance company for review, s/he may not be a specialist for that treatment plan, so a true peer-to-peer discussion does not occur.

It gets even trickier when insurance guidelines don't match the specialty medical society recommendations. For example, a family physician may review an endocrinologist's request for re-imaging an adrenal mass. The insurance company may limit re-imaging to once a year, whereas the American Association of Clinical Endocrinologists (AACE) guidelines recommend re-imaging every 3-6 months.

This administrative burden distracts physicians from practicing medicine and contributes to burnout. In response, practices must add or shift staff just to deal with prior auths. One study estimated that, on average, prior authorization requests consumed about 20 hours a week per medical practice. This included one hour of the doctor's time, nearly six hours of clerical time, plus 13 hours of nurses' time. Another study by Health Affairs further revealed practices spent an average of $68,274 per physician per year interacting with health plans, equating to $31 billion annually. In a recent MGMA survey, 90% of health care leaders noted an increase in prior authorization requirements in 2019   . It's not getting better. Projections show prior authorization for prescription drugs will increase 20% per year.

What complicates matters is that even if the insurance allows the request, it does not guarantee payment. It also does not ensure the patient will be eligible on the date of service. To top it off, the insurance company may still conduct a post-payment review to verify medical necessity. In some situations, prior authorization isn't determined until after the treatment is complete. For example, a patient may be hospitalized 3 days for pneumonia. After being discharged, the insurance may decide that the patient should have only been hospitalized under an observation admission, which is less than 48 hours. When this happens, the insurance company will hold some or all the expected payment to the physician. This leaves the physician chasing after the patient for payment, often writing off the charges as bad debt.

Who Loses?

In the end, it's the patients who lose the most from the pre-auth process. According to an AMA survey, 75% of physicians reported issues related to the prior authorization process can cause patients to abandon their recommended course of treatment. What's more alarming is 28% of physicians reported pre-auth delays led to a serious adverse event for a patient in their care.

Another study examined the records of over 4,000 patients with type 2 diabetes who were prescribed medications requiring prior authorizations. Those denied the medications had higher overall medical costs during the following year. Therefore, it cost insurers more in the long term as they seek other treatment and medication. Patients who can no longer wait for an authorization seek treatment at an emergency room or urgent care facility, which is often not covered by their health plan. On those occasions, the insurance company saves money, but they shift the cost to the patients.

How to fix Prior Authorizations

To fix prior authorizations, we should shift the approval process from those providing the care to the insurance company requiring approval. We can begin by exempting physicians with a demonstrated approval record from many prior authorization requirements. Texas is doing this now by "gold carding" physicians who have a 90% prior authorization approval rate over a 6-month period on certain services. Gold carded physicians are exempt from prior authorization requirements for those services, so state-regulated insurance companies will not delay patient care.

We also need to stop requiring prior authorizations for preventive care services that are state-mandated, like mammograms and colonoscopy screenings. We should require insurance plans to inform patients and physicians of their pre-auth policies.

In addition, requests need to be reviewed by physicians who practice in the same or similar specialty. We should also require all insurance companies to create directories that clearly identify specialty physicians and facilities that are in-network.

Insurers should use standard electronic prior authorization (ePA) that automates authorizations by integrating with the EHR, making the process faster, consistent across insurers, and more efficient. Unfortunately, health plans currently offering ePA options require physicians or their staff to log into their site and use their proprietary portals. This means exiting the EHR, re-entering clinical data, and then logging back into the EHR afterward.

States and medical organizations understand the negative effect prior authorizations have on patient care. The AMA has partnered with over 50 medical organizations to urge health plans and utilization review entities to apply 21 principles to utilization management programs for both medical and pharmacy benefits. I paraphrased a few of them below:

- Utilization management programs should allow for flexibility, including the timely overriding of step therapy requirements. Step therapy requires patients to try one or more medications specified by the insurance company, usually less expensive, to treat a health condition. The patient has to fail this medication before being allowed to "step up" to another medicine or treatment that may be more expensive.
- If a patient switches health plans, the new plan should not require patients to repeat step therapy protocols before qualifying for coverage of a current effective therapy.
- Once approved, the utilization review entity should not revoke, limit, condition, or restrict coverage for authorized care provided within 45 business days from the date authorization was received.

We need to refocus on patient care and let physicians practice medicine. Until then, we'll continue to see physicians distracted from clinical care and increasing percentages of physician burnout. The unstructured and unpredictable nature of prior authorizations can destroy daily clinical workflows and negatively impact patient care.

DOC RELATED

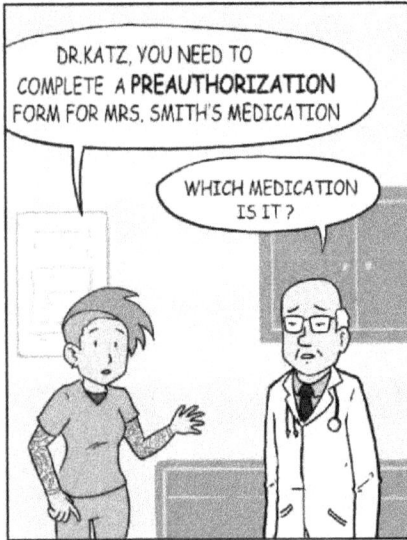

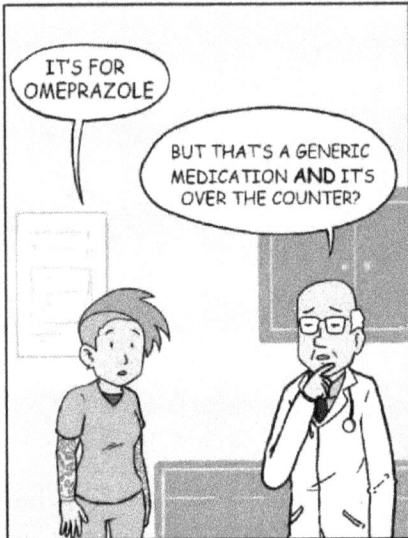

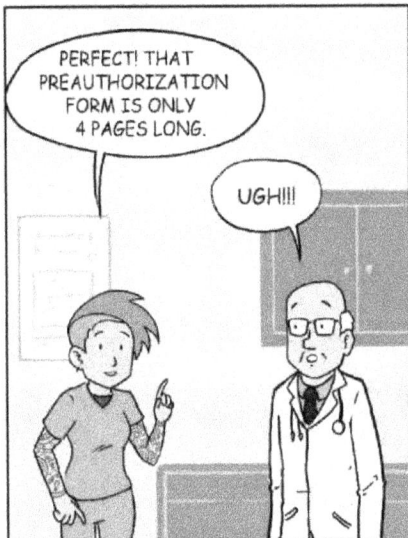

Dr. Peter Valenzuela

DOC ☞ RELATED

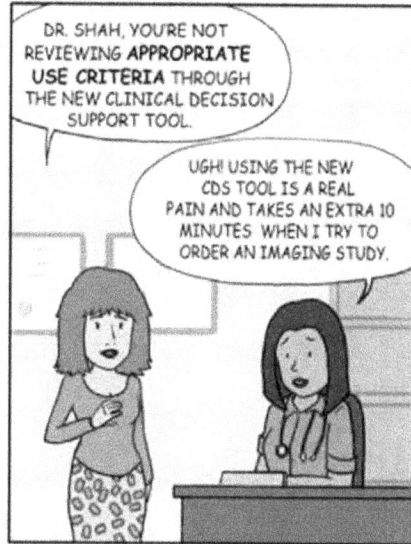

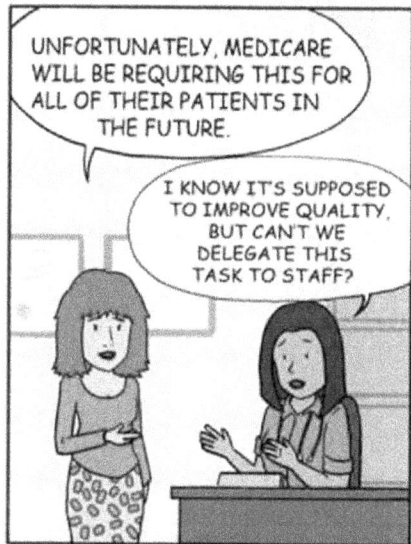

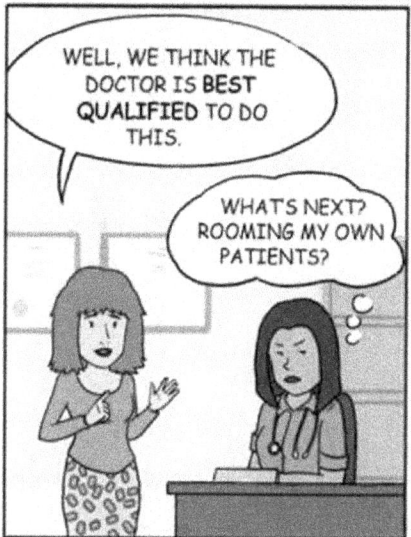

Dr. Peter Valenzuela

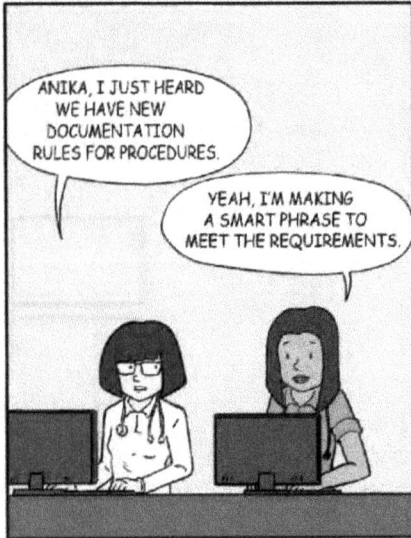

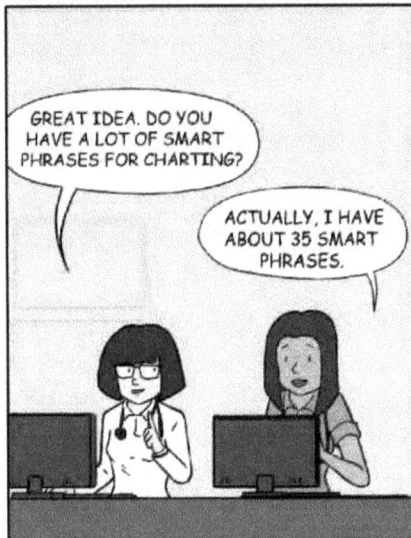

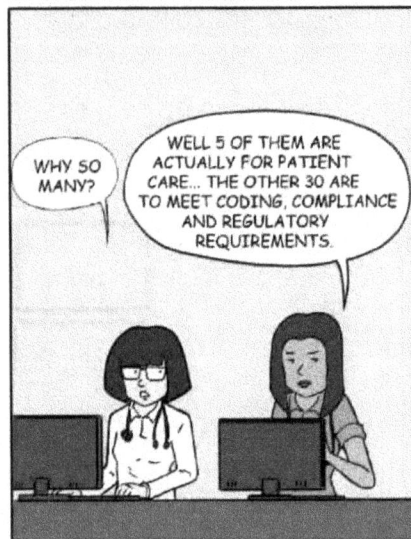

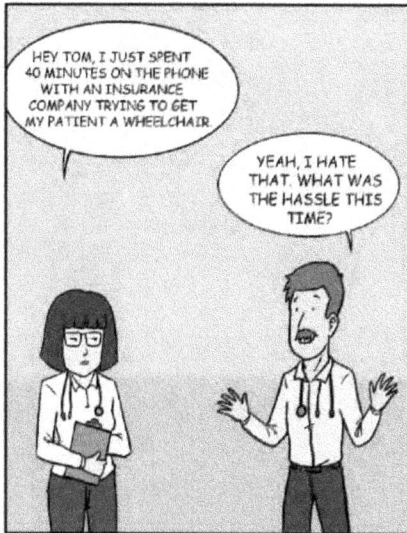

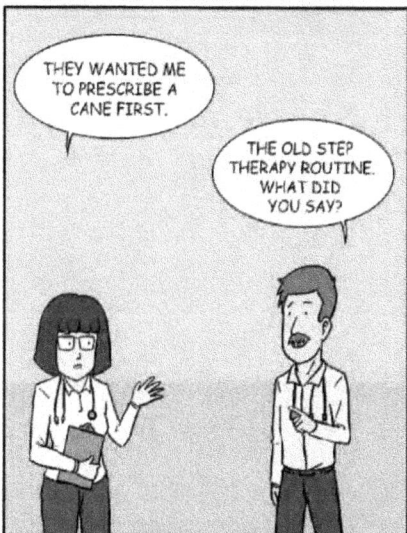

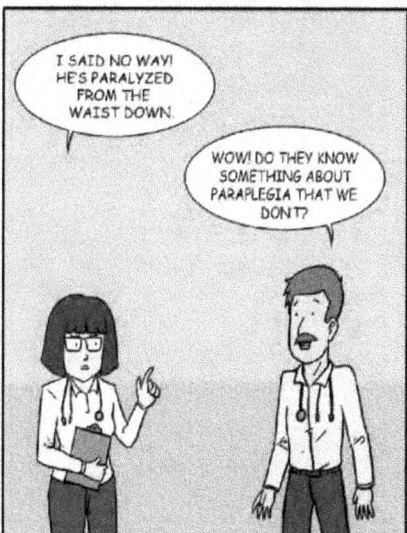

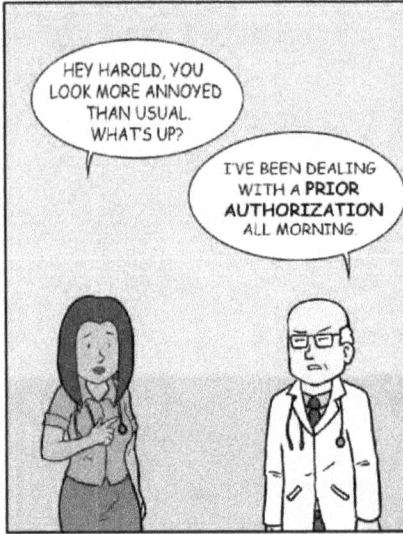

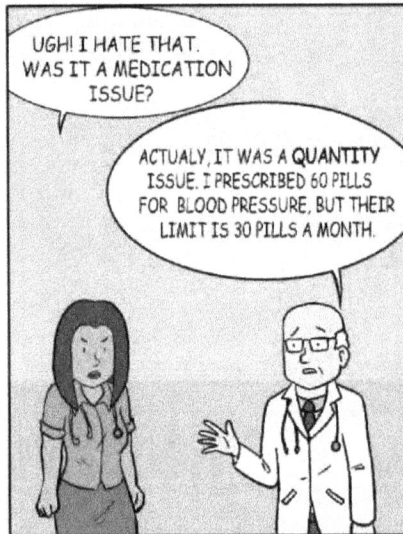

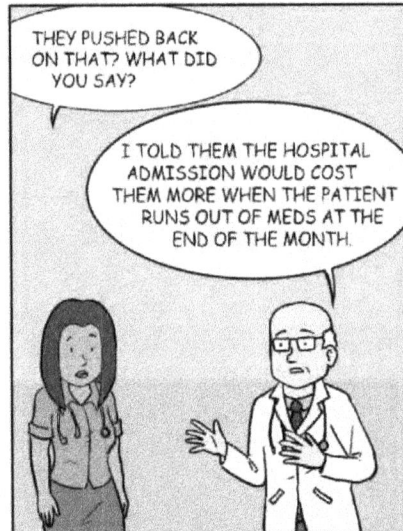

Chapter 7
Coding: What's The Code for That?

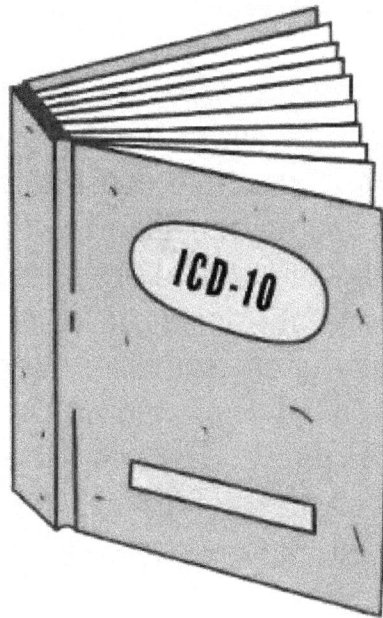

Like pre-auths, coding is causing all kinds of pain points for physicians, support staff, and patients. The original health care coding system began in 17th century England. They gathered statistical data through a system known as the London Bills of Mortality and arranged it into numerical codes.

These codes were used to measure the most frequent causes of death. In 1937, they organized this statistical analysis of the causes of death into the International List of Causes of Death.

Over the years, the World Health Organization (WHO) used this list more and more to help track mortality rates and international health trends. The list was later developed into the International Classification of Diseases (ICD), which is now in its 10th edition (ICD-10). In 1977, they expanded the ICD system to not only include causes of death but also clinical diagnoses such as illnesses and injuries. Adding clinical diagnoses provided additional statistical information on basic healthcare.

Understanding Coding Complexity

Evaluation and management (E/M) coding is how physicians and clinicians translate patient encounters into five-digit current procedural terminology (CPT) codes for billing. Every billable procedure has its own individual CPT code. There are different E/M codes for different encounters, such as office visits or hospital visits. Within each type of encounter, there are different levels of care. Each patient care encounter requires specific documentation based on three "key" components: history, physical exam, medical decision-Making.

The Centers for Medicare and Medicaid Services (CMS) developed the E/M guidelines in partnership with the American Medical Association (AMA). Higher paying E/M codes (like consultations or initial office visits) require more extensive documentation than lower-paying codes (like office visits with established patients or hospital progress notes).

In following these rules, physicians have to consider multiple factors when selecting codes. First, where was the service performed? Was it done in the clinic, hospital, emergency room, ambulatory surgery center, nursing home, patient's home, or virtually? If done virtually, was it a video visit, telephone encounter, or online messaging?

Second, who performed the service? Was it done by the physician directly? Was it done by someone working under the physician's supervision, like an advanced practice clinician, resident physician, nurse, or medical assistant? Third, was the patient seen for multiple conditions? If so, which condition should be listed first, second, etc.? Fourth, were multiple services performed? For example, did you treat the person for a concussion and stitch them up for a head laceration from the fall? If you performed multiple services, what modifier code should be selected?

Last, how long did you spend with the patient? Should a time-based code be selected? Every one of these components is vital because it decides whether an encounter will be paid and how much the insurer will pay the provider. Now imagine being a health care professional with 15 minutes to see the patient AND chart AND code.

Years ago in Washington State, I worked with Dr. Warren Taranow, an orthopedic surgeon who was extremely focused on his coding. He kept a short list of common orthopedic codes taped to his office wall. He also used a CD-ROM with procedure codes from the American Academy of Orthopedic Surgeons. Not to be caught short on resources, he kept an ICD-9 book on his shelf. As the head of the medical group, I admired his dedication and how well he captured codes. Back then, there were already an unmanageable 13,000 ICD-9 codes. Today, we have approximately 70,000 ICD-10 codes in health care, with over 400 diagnosis codes associated with diabetes alone!

Not only is the coding process complicated, but it's also comical. Dr. Halee Fischer Wright provides hilarious insights into the insanity of codes in her book *Back to Balance*, where she asks readers to answer whether a code is actual or a way Kenny, a fictional character in the animated South Park series, is killed. Being an art buff, I also found a splendid book titled *Struck by Orca* published by ICD-10 Illustrated that incorporates outrageous codes with illustrated depictions. Just in case you're wondering, the actual ICD-10 code for being struck by an orca is W56.22xA.

HCC and RAF Scores

There is increasing momentum for value-based care, which should lower health care costs and better outcomes for patients. One way it does this is by strengthening payor cost controls and reducing their risk. I mentioned that there are approximately 70,000 ICD-10 codes. Over 9,500 of them map to the 86 Hierarchical Condition Categories (HCC) used by Medicare for value-based payments. HCC coding is used to assign patients a Risk Adjust Factor (RAF) score to better describe patient complexity. The sicker the patient, the higher the RAF score.

Despite the cumbersome and confusing process, clinicians are responsible for ensuring that they properly capture HCC and RAF codes. On the plus side, coding order of diagnosis, site of service, or provider type are not factored into the HCC algorithm. However, they are factored into the other 60,000 non-HCC mapped codes, so it's hard for docs to distinguish unless they're made aware by staff. HCC coding is hard for physicians because it does nothing to change the treatment plan. It's just part of the song and dance of getting paid. Unfortunately, coding education is rarely a priority during medical school and residency training, so it can prove overwhelming for physicians and clinicians when they join a practice.

Who's Responsible for Coding?

Health care professionals sign agreements with payors attesting those accurate claims will be submitted. According to CMS, "A billing specialist or alternate source may review the provider's documented services before submitting the claim to a payer. These reviewers may help select codes that best reflect the provider's furnished services."

The problem is that not all physicians and organizations use coders. Those that do may have them serving more in auditing roles for fear of financial penalties for inappropriate coding. Those that don't have any coders put the responsibility on the backs of clinicians.

Ways to Fix Coding

Every minute a physician spends doing non-clinical work is detrimental to patient care and the joy of their work. As Dr. Dike Drummond, aka the HappyMD, states, "Coders should code, billers should bill, and doctors should see patients" I've practiced medicine for 20 years. I can honestly say that I welcome coding support and would happily hand it over to a coder, so I can focus on things that matter to me.

Although administration may argue that having dedicated medical coders is cost-prohibitive, they more than pay for themselves. Just one HCC coder with the right charge review automation software can improve RAF accuracy by 20%, resulting in more Medicare savings. Coders are also vital in preventing denials. Every denial cost practices $25 to $30 each to work.

Along with coders, we should leverage technology to assist or perform the coding. Platforms currently exist that use artificial intelligence to reduce errors in medical coding as well as predict and suggest ICD-10 and CPT codes based on text, images, and reports from the patient encounter.

Last, we need to simplify the coding process. This means eliminating the coding and documentation requirements that consume so much time. In 2021, CMS changed the documentation requirements that no longer require a history and exam to select an E/M service, but it still must be performed in order to report certain CPT codes. We now base code selection on either level of medical decision-making or time performing the service on the day of the encounter.

This is a step in the right direction, but we'll have to see how it is rolled out and monitored. Unfortunately, other payers have not committed to this type of coding, so physicians still must document differently for different payers. Also, the change only applies to five ambulatory-based E/M Codes, not consultations or hospital visits.

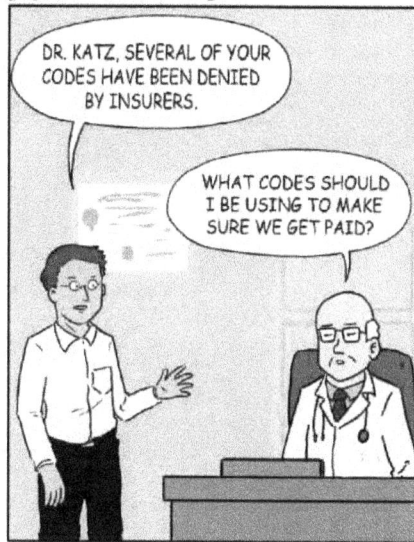

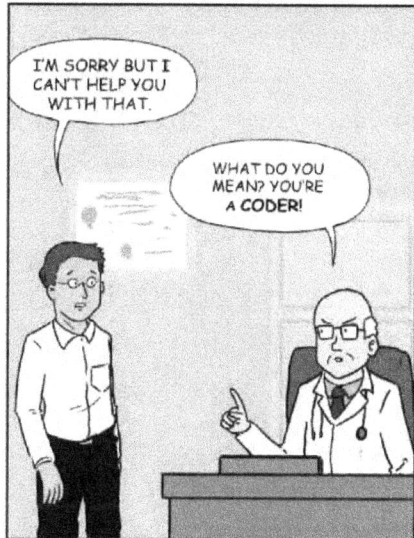

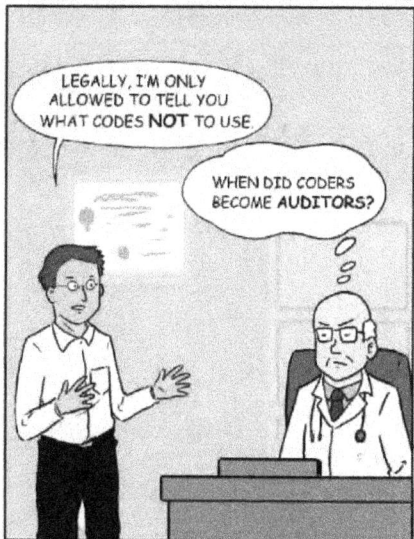

DOC RELATED

CHIP, I DEMAND A CODER! I'M SPENDING ALL MY TIME LOOKING UP ICD-10 CODES!

I WISH I COULD HELP YOU HAROLD BUT CORPORATE POLICY STATES THAT PHYSICIANS ARE RESPONSIBLE FOR THEIR OWN CODING.

I'M ALSO RESPONSIBLE FOR MY OWN TAXES BUT I HAVE AN ACCOUNTANT DO THEM FOR ME.

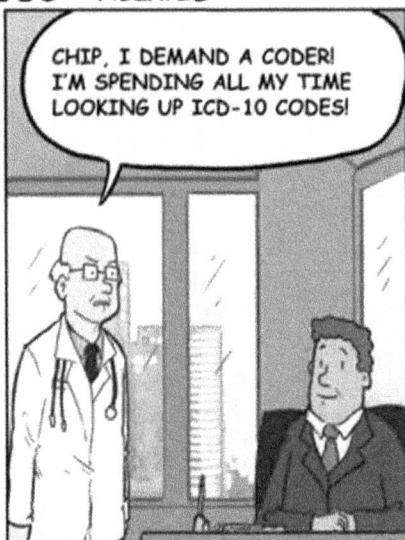

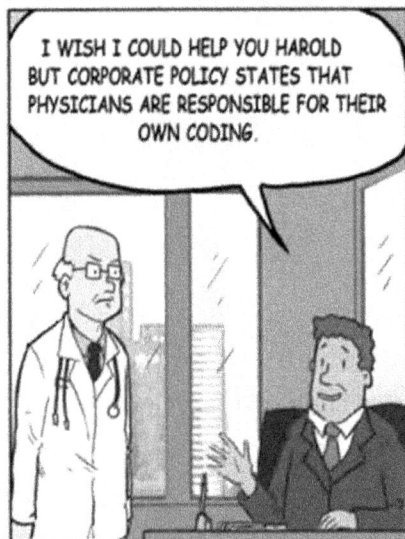

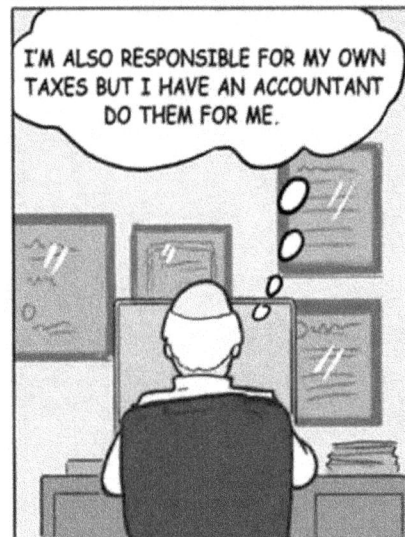

Dr .Peter Valenzuela

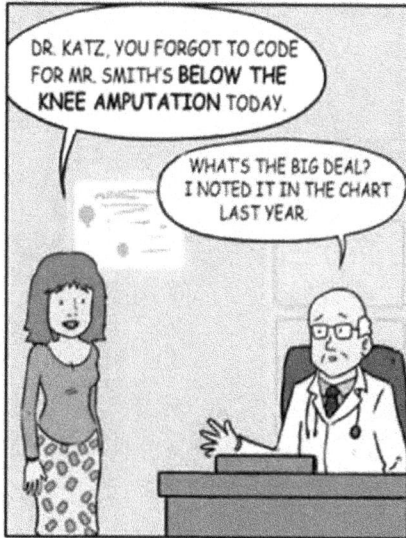

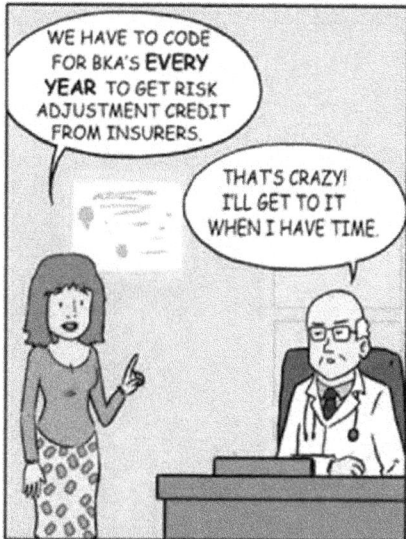

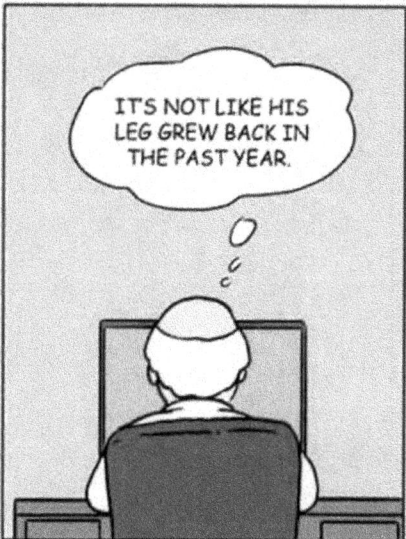

DOC RELATED

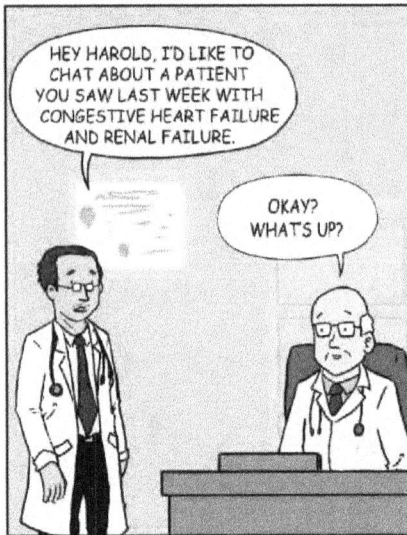

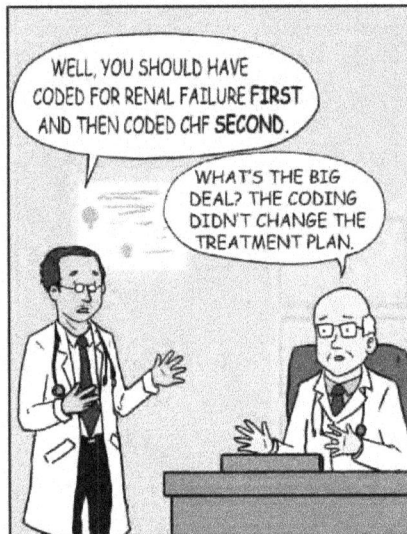

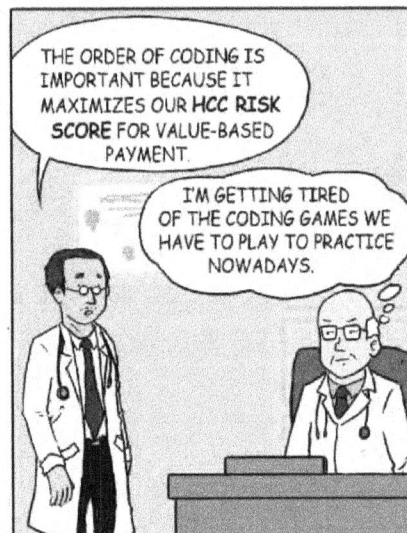

Dr. Peter Valenzuela

Chapter 8
Physician Productivity: Squeeze in More Patients

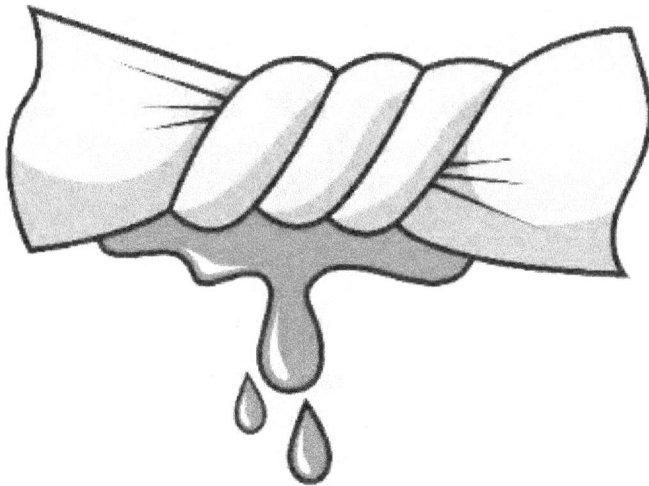

If you ask a doctor for the best jokes they can remember, they will probably be self-deprecating or insults about their colleagues. One of the most common jokes I remember from med school is called, "How do you hide $100 from a doctor?" It goes something like this:

How do you hide $100 from an orthopedic surgeon? Stick it to a stethoscope.

How do you hide $100 from a general surgeon? Tape it to the patient's notes

How do you hide $100 from a radiologist? Tape it to a patient.

How do you hide $100 from a cardiologist? That's a trick question. You can't.

How do you hide $100 from a family doctor? Don't worry, they don't know what $100 bill looks like.

Although meant to be playful banter among physicians, it holds some level of truth based on the specialty chosen and how much they are paid. Proceduralists — like surgeons and cardiologists — are paid substantially higher than primary care physicians. To better understand how physicians are paid, you must know how work is measured and rewarded in health care.

How Work is Measured.

We call the standard metric for work a relative value unit (RVU). CMS established it, and it determines the amount to pay doctors, providers, and suppliers based on their productivity. It includes work performed for over 10,000 procedures and services covered under the CMS Physician Fee Schedule. Private insurers also use this fee schedule to set their rates with providers. There are three types of RVUs:

1.   **Physician work RVUs** account for the time, technical skill and effort, mental effort and judgment, and stress to provide a service. The work RVU makes up around 53 percent of the total RVU across all procedures with RVU values.
2.   **Practice expense RVUs** account for the nonphysician clinical and non-clinical labor of the practice, as well as expenses for building space, equipment, and office supplies.
3.   **Professional liability insurance RVUs** account for the cost of malpractice insurance premiums. Although the actual percentages vary from service to service, physician work and practice expenses comprise 52 and 44 percent of total Medicare expenditures on physician services, respectively.

The calculation for total RVUs includes these three components and a geographic adjustment factor (GAF) for each. To get the total RVUS, you add all three together. CMS adds geographic adjustments because performing a procedure in one region, like California, with higher labor and facility costs, may be more expensive than in another region, like Texas. They base GAF on the geographic practice cost index (GPCI).

A major component of the RVU is the service code, which is provided by the AMA. The lower the service code, the less the intensity of work credited by the AMA's service code, and the less pay. This is where things get challenging. CMS pays physicians 3 to 5 times more for common procedural care than for cognitive care . Therefore, specialists who perform procedures or services in the hospital or surgery center are paid more. This method is a major frustration for non-procedural specialists.

For example, an office visit by an internist for a new patient with congestive heart failure, high cholesterol, and diabetes may take an hour to perform after reviewing records, imaging, patient history, examination, and discussion with the patient. This one-hour-plus visit might generate 3.17 RVUs for the physician. During that same timeframe, a gastroenterologist can perform three straightforward colonoscopies with a polypectomy and earn 14 RVUs. This is not to detract from the gastroenterologist's work, but to say that non-procedural physicians also have high-intensity encounters that are not properly credited.

Adding to the Frustration

CMS relies on advice and recommendations from the AMA's Specialty Society Relative Value Scale Update Committee (RUC) to determine RVU values. The members of RUC include those recognized by the American Board of Medical Specialties, those with a large percentage of physicians in patient care, and those that account for high percentages of Medicare expenditures. The RUC also includes four seats that rotate on a two-year basis, with two reserved for an internal medicine subspecialty, one for a primary care representative, and one for any other specialty.

Here's where it gets complicated: for valuing work, it's a zero-sum game. Increasing the RVUs for any service will cause a commensurate decrease in fees for other physician services. This leads to "horizontal hostility," pitting physicians against each other to validate their worth in RVUs. Historically, higher RVU credit has highly depended on the compositions of the RUC, making it a political game.

Why Healthcare Organizations Partner with Docs

Remember from the chapter on insurance that managed care programs do not use RVUs the same way. They focus on risk-based agreements paying monthly per-member payments. However, since health care is still 70% fee-for-service, it behooves organizations to hire or partner with proceduralists to maximize revenue. Understanding that these proceduralists need a referral base, organizations also acquire or partner with primary care doctors.

As physicians increasingly join or incorporate into hospital organizations, RVUs are the standard measure for physician productivity used to calculate physician compensation. On the plus side, the RVU system removes doctors' risk relative to employer-negotiated payments, reductions in reimbursement, or collection problems. On the negative side, this RVU model can overwhelm newly employed doctors who previously controlled their own schedules and could spend extra time with patients when needed. That's why productivity targets are a key driver of physician burnout.

Here's the irony: although almost half of physicians believe fee-for-service is more expensive for health care costs, a 2015 study revealed that 73% of physicians prefer this model of payment. Physicians aren't convinced that value-based models actually improve clinical outcomes. We'll talk more about value metrics in the next section.

Since then, we've gone through a pandemic that poked multiple holes in the productivity model. In August 2020, physicians reported an average drop in revenue of 32% since February 2020. About one in five doctors saw revenue drop by 50% or more, while nearly one-third saw declines of between 25% and 49%. Only 19% of physicians reported no drop in revenue.

How it Affects Patients

The straight RVU model of compensation rewards doctors for seeing more patients, regardless of outcomes or patient satisfaction. Physicians who are more thoughtful and thorough in their approach are penalized, even if the outcomes are better. Spending more time with patients addressing all their concerns produces only a limited amount of RVUs. Working under a strictly RVU model may also encourage overutilization of tests and procedures, which can decrease the quality of care and lead to unnecessary health care costs.

Ways to Fix How Work is Measured

In chapter five, I discussed how changing the insurance payment model will ultimately change the way we compensate physicians. Moving towards a single-payer or advanced payments will allow more creativity in modeling for physicians. Until then, one of the quickest ways to right-size the RVU gap is to increase the value for services requiring higher levels of cognitive thinking to help prevent illness.

In 2021, CMS did just that. They took active measures to value cognitive specialists for their time and effort by increasing RVU credit for ambulatory-based codes. At the same time, CMS lowered the conversion factor that is multiplied by the RVU. A few of the specialty winners included endocrinologists, rheumatologists, oncologists, and primary care doctors. However, because it's a zero-sum game, a few of the losers included anesthesiologists, cardiac surgeons, interventional radiologists, and thoracic surgeons.

Although this does level-set the traditional inequities in work based on time and effort, it still relies on RVUs to measure the work. Another way to fix the RVU productivity model is to change the way we compensate physicians. Doctors and clinicians should receive more of a base salary with upside potential for non-RVU categories like citizenship, patient growth, quality outcomes, and practice financial performance. Citizenship may include activities that advance the organization, including participation in committees, community service, lean events, and variation reduction projects.

The good news is that between 2012 and 2018, the percentage of physicians paid by a productivity-only model dropped from 51.8 percent to 42.7 percent. However, much of these changes occurred in ambulatory-based doctors, with most proceduralists still being paid on predominantly production models. Understanding that most health care organizations are still predominantly fee-for-service, the ultimate driver of change will be the payers moving to more value-based agreements.

DOC ⬤ RELATED

Panel 1:
OVER HERE IS OUR SPECIALTY CLINIC.
WHO'S THAT?

Panel 2:
THAT'S DR. BERRY.
WHY IS HE WEARING A SUPERHERO CAPE?

Panel 3:
BECAUSE HE'S A SURGEON.
OH, THAT MAKES **TOTAL SENSE** NOW.

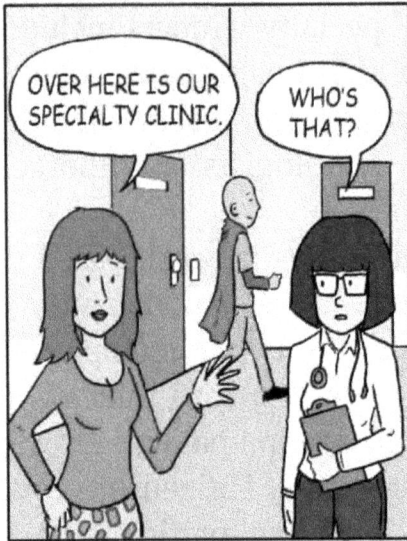

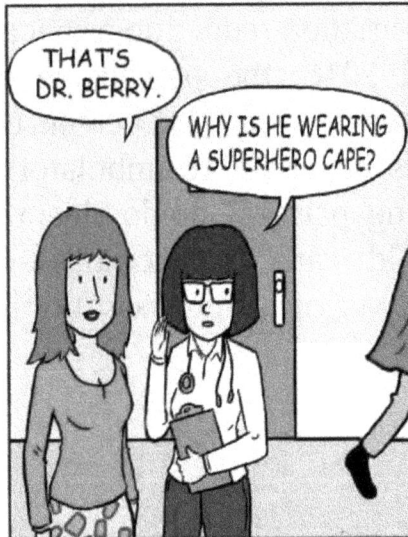

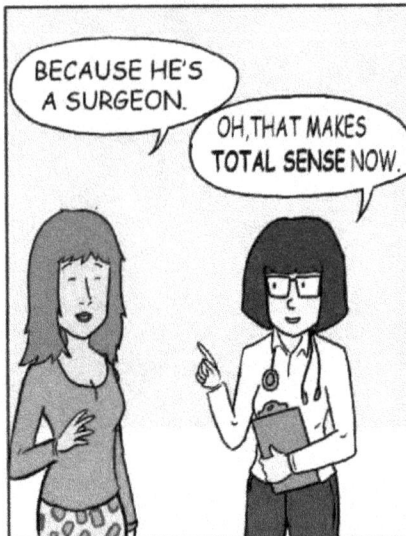

Dr. Peter Valenzuela

DOC-RELATED

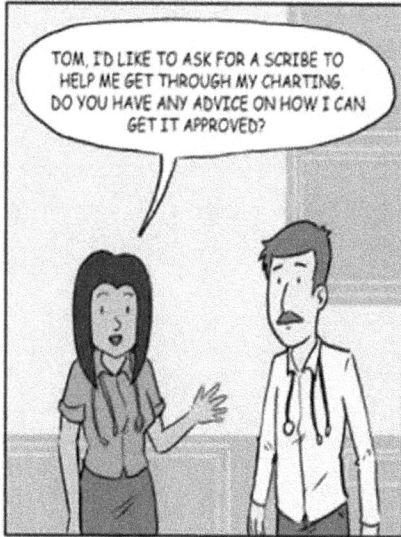

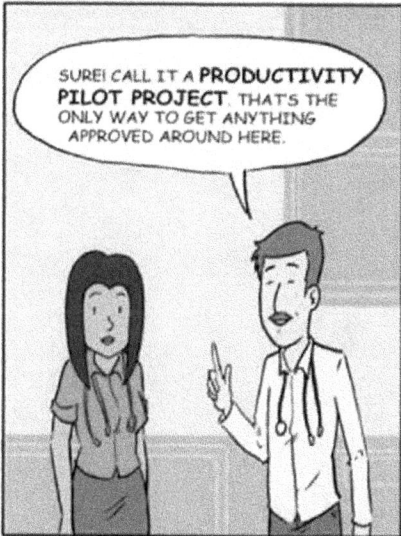

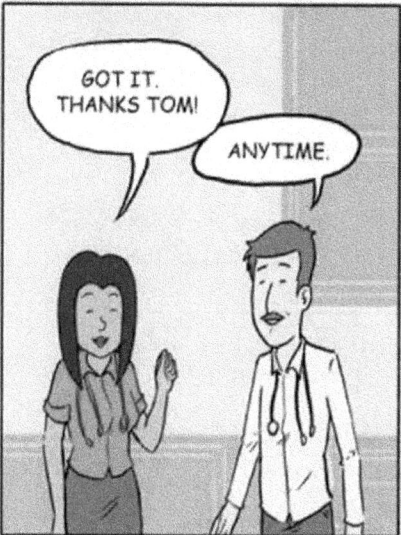

Dr. Peter Valenzuela

DOC·RELATED

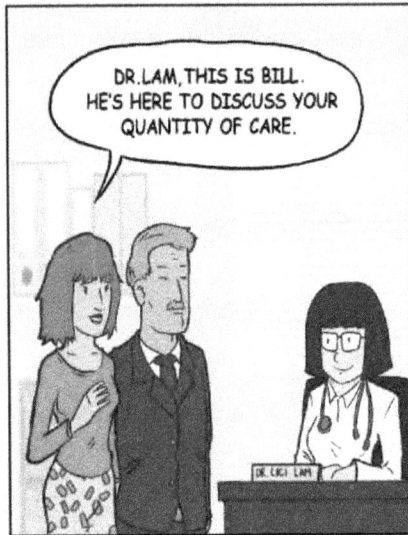

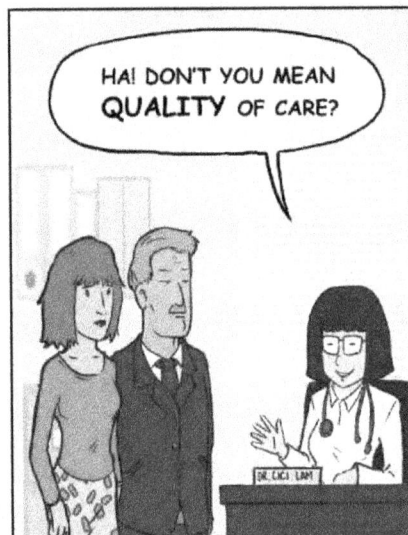

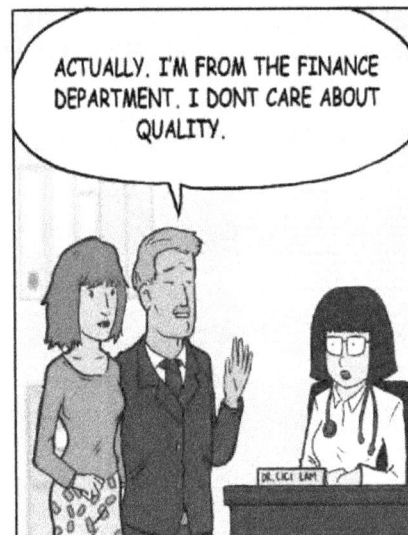

Dr. Peter Valenzuela

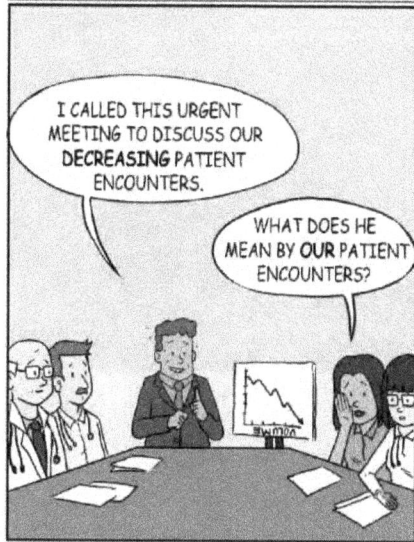

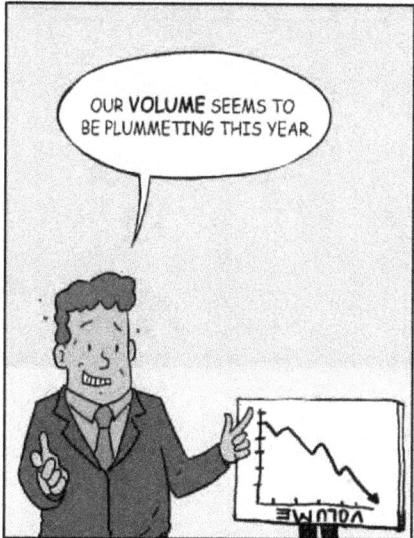

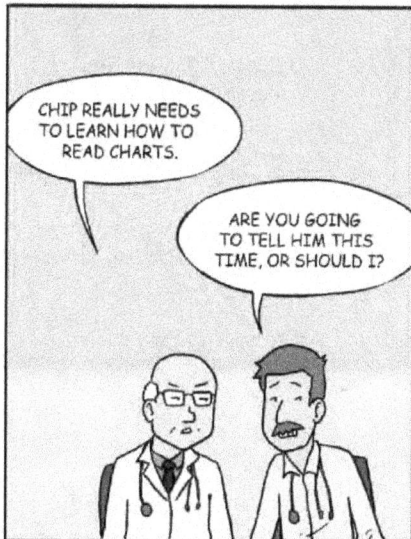

DOC RELATED

Panel 1: GREAT NEWS DR. SHAH! OUR PERFORMANCE IMPROVEMENT TEAM HAS FOUND A WAY TO ADD 3 MORE PATIENTS INTO YOUR SCHEDULE BEFORE 5 PM.

Panel 2: BUT DONNA, EACH PATIENT I SEE MEANS MORE TIME SPENT CHARTING FOR ME AFTER 5 PM.

Panel 3: UNFORTUNATELY, OUR PERFORMANCE IMPROVEMENT TEAM DOESN'T WORK AFTER 5 PM. YOU'LL HAVE TO SOLVE THAT PROBLEM ON YOUR OWN.

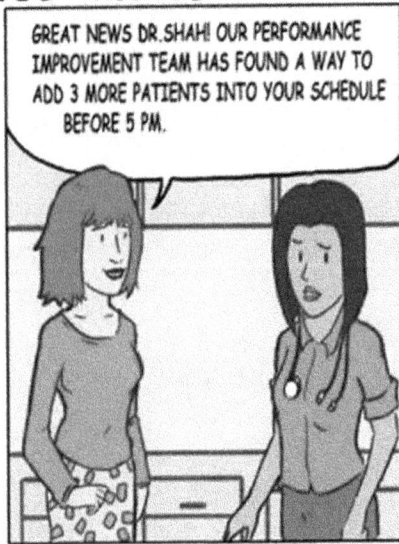

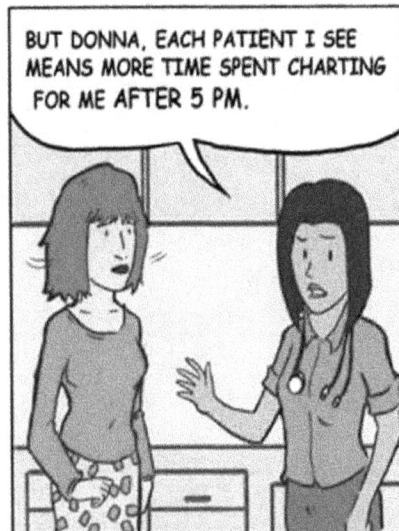

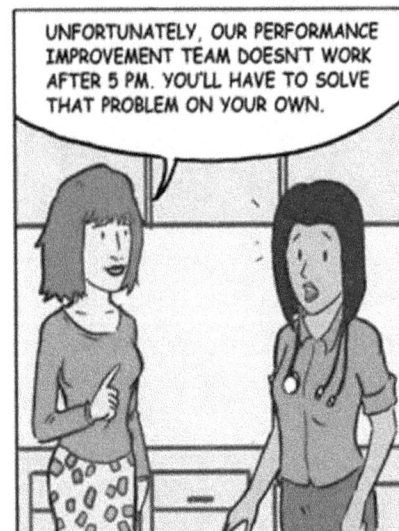

Dr. Peter Valenzuela

Part 3:
Charting & Regulations

Chapter 9
Electronic Health Records: Charting to Infinity

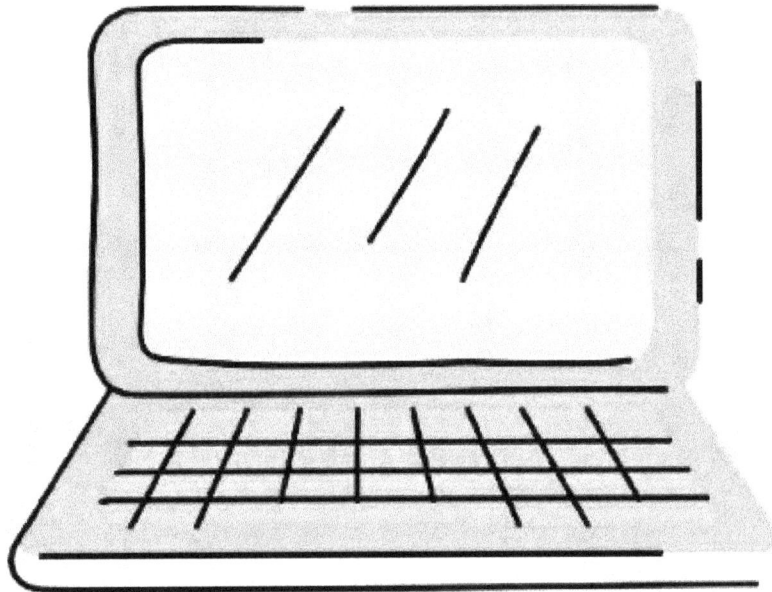

In March 2019, a physician created a Twitter account to mock one of the biggest EHR giants in the industry. The account quickly gained 22,000 followers and was featured in multiple publications. Like Dr. Glaucomflecken, the physician account holder posted in anonymity due to fear of retribution by the vendor and his employer. All posts parodied the evil voice of the EHR software's leadership.

In his description, he wrote, "My goal is to create confusion for doctors. I will not rest until doctors do nothing but click buttons. Eye contact is evil." To be clear, the EHR company had nothing to do with this account, but I'm pretty sure they disliked it. The primary message this physician expressed in his posts was that EHRs take up so much of the doctor's attention that the patient-doctor relationship suffers. A few of my favorite posts included:

(EHR vendor) doesn't take a day off. So why should you? Your (EHR vendor) inbox fills up 365 days per year, and you need to be there to empty it. Remember our motto: Turn Free Time Into (EHR) Time.

After a study showed surgery residents spend nearly 8 months of their 5-Year Training in the Electronic Health Record, this account posted:

I'm proud of this, but it shows I have work to do. 8 months is not enough.

After a physician posted, "Minutes ago, I finished 28 years of education and training. Gratitude is the feeling of the moment." The account posted:

Should I ruin this by letting him know what's in his future?

Satire aside, EHRs have a tremendous mental and emotional impact on physicians. When I first started working as a chief medical officer, I rounded on the care centers regularly. During that time, I tried to get quick wins to improve the working environment for our docs and staff. Some wins were relatively easy, like replacing the coffeemaker in the lounge or having tech support set up printers closer to clinical workstations.

One day, I stopped to chat with Larry, a family physician who was in the twilight of his career. When I asked him how it was going, he looked at me exasperated and said, "Peter, I've been trying to figure out how to order a vaccine for my patient for the last 20 minutes!" Once we finally figured out how to order the vaccine, Larry looked at me and said, "This just isn't fun anymore. I spend so much time charting that I don't get to spend time with my patients or to chat in the hallway with my colleagues like I used to in the old days." Larry is an extrovert who enjoys mentoring and helping others. It was heartbreaking to hear, but not an unfamiliar story. Many doctors today are suffering from social isolation as doctor-patient relationships and relationships among colleagues suffer due to time constraints.

Martin Seligman, a positive psychology guru, outlined the fundamental ingredients needed to achieve happiness and well-being in his book *Flourish*. Using an acronym, PERMA, his building blocks include Positive emotions, Engagement, Relationships, Meaning, and Accomplishment . These were the components missing in Larry's work — and many physicians like him whose lives revolve around electronic health records. Pre-EHR, docs spent more time curb-siding with each other and joking with the staff. (Curb-siding is asking another colleague for their medical advice related to a patient.)

There was a sense of community, and people looked forward to coming to work. Post-EHR, people became more disconnected and less likely to help one another. I'm not saying having fun at work isn't occurring at all anymore, but it may not be as frequent.

Where Does the Time Go?

During an 11.4-hour workday, doctors spend 5.1 hours with patients and spend 5.9 hours in the EHR . Roughly 25% of that computer work happens after clinic hours. The annual cost of physicians spending half of their time using EHRs is over $365 billion (a billion dollars per day) — more than the United States spends treating any major class of diseases and about equal to what the country spends on public primary and secondary education instruction.

Why do we Spend so Much Time Charting?

Twenty years ago, I used paper charts to document my notes. I had the option to dictate, but my handwriting was legible enough for staff and clinicians to understand my diagnoses and follow-up plan for the patient. My notes met E/M documentation requirements with aspects of history, physical exam, and medical decision-making. Back then, I could see up to 35 patients a day and not feel overwhelmed. I was technically savvy and used a secure app on my phone to prescribe medications and print them out for patients digitally. My notes were much shorter and more relevant to anyone who read them. They told a story about the patient and helped others understand what I was thinking. Below is a typical note for a diabetic patient visit I would have written when I started practice in 2001:

SUBJECTIVE: Mrs. X is a 42-year-old Hispanic female with diabetes. Her blood sugars have been running in the low 200s at home. She admits to not complying with her diet ever since her mom moved in and has been cooking lots of high-carb foods. Patient denies polydipsia, polyuria, or visual changes. No numbness to extremities.

OBJECTIVE: BP 127/79. Blood sugar today is 207 fasting. Overweight Hispanic female in no distress.

ASSESSMENT: Poorly controlled diabetes

PLAN: I advised the patient to continue Metformin 500 mg twice a day. Add glyburide 5 mg daily. Monitor sugars daily and follow up in 2 weeks.

Unfortunately, EHRs have shifted our focus less on communicating care plans to share with colleagues to document for the powers that control our payment. Compared to other countries using the same EHR, clinical notes in the United States are nearly 4 times longer on average than those in other countries . These countries have something we don't — universal health care. With all patients being insured, physicians there focus more on the care of the patient and less on how the encounter will be paid. They are exempt from the highly regulated coding and charting requirements we face in the U.S.

EHRs have some benefits. They have made our notes more legible. They've also made it easier to comply with all the billing and regulatory mandates, which seem to be the core function of EHRs. EHR features allow physicians to copy previous notes and paste them on a current note. We can also use "smart sets" and "dot phrases" to create one-size-fits-all templates and auto-populate information for every encounter. But using dot phrases and copy-paste can create another problem — extremely bloated notes with unnecessary information.

In all transparency, I never read all the notes from other physicians about my patients anymore because it would take way too much time. Instead, I look at the assessment and plan to see what needs to be done. EHRs have removed much of the art and personalization out of medicine. For physicians, what was once telling a story about a patient has become more like an automated transaction with a widget. Even if a physician wished to stay true to the art of medicine and dictate their note outside of the EHR, the document would just be scanned into the platform and placed in a miscellaneous section of the chart, where it's unlikely to be discovered or read again.

Interoperability

One would think that moving to electronic health records would make the availability of data much easier, which was a goal of the Health Information Technology for Economic and Clinical Health (HITECH) Act passed in 2009. Unfortunately, this never materialized because officials allowed hundreds of competing companies to sell EHR software that couldn't exchange information. This oversight has made patient information difficult to access, or it spreads information out in multiple systems, wasting time physicians could spend with patients.

At a meeting with health care leaders in 2017, then Vice President Joe

Biden talked about how difficult it was to get his son's records from one hospital to another. "I was stunned when my son for a year was battling stage 4 glioblastoma. I couldn't get his records. I'm the Vice President of the United States of America.... It was an absolute nightmare. It was ridiculous, absolutely ridiculous, that we're in that circumstance."

Like everything else, interoperability depends on profits for vendors who worry that record-sharing will lead to a loss in market share. Health care organizations market ease of information exchange within their integrated delivery network to attract payers and patients. Vendors try to make it too expensive or too technically difficult to migrate to another EHR. The result is more paperwork for staff who must manually scan documents into the EHR system. Even then, the data goes into miscellaneous folders that cannot be queried and takes exorbitant amounts of time for physicians to review.

Dealing with the Inbox

Now that we've touched on charting and lack of interoperability, let's talk about another EHR frustration for physicians — the infamous inbox. This is the work that happens between patient encounters and often at night. Physicians spend approximately 25% of their work time in the inbox. Responsibilities can include patient calls, patient messages, prescription refills, relaying lab and test results, insurance and other forms, and doctor to doctor consults, to name a few. Physicians average 243 inbox messages per week. Some primary care and medical specialties have hundreds of items in multiple buckets on a weekly basis.

I previously worked with a family physician who averaged eight hours of "pajama time" every day! Although the term sounds fun, pajama time is a measure of the time physicians spend doing administrative work outside regular clinic hours. She was essentially working two jobs, but only getting paid for one. Like many docs, she could never turn off the work switch and felt morally obligated to finish every task by the end of the day so patient care would not suffer. In the end, she resigned from the group, feeling overwhelmed and unable to keep up with the pace of virtual care work. As if a physician's self-motivation is not enough, many organizations have financial penalties for physicians who don't complete their in-box work in a timely fashion.

How to Fix the EHR

Roughly two-thirds of primary care physicians think EHRs have led to improved care, but six out of 10 physicians think EHRs need a complete overhaul. Like any product, the goal of EHRs should be to target the user experience. The first step we should take to enhance the user experience is to remove the number of clicks needed to do the work by following a mantra of removing a click for every click added. We can apply lean techniques, like process mapping, to shadow clinicians throughout their day and identify non-value-added work. We should also identify the ideal person to complete tasks, so all members of the clinical team are working at the top of their license. Not all tasks — like medication refills and normal lab reviews — need to be completed by a physician.

Besides workflows and working at the top of licensure, we should incorporate different ways to document to offload time spent charting and allow physicians to focus on patient care. Documentation options could include voice recognition software and scribes — live or virtual. Another option is to incorporate artificial intelligence-supported technologies like computer-assisted physician documentation (CAPD), which show improvements in patient care by ensuring accurate, complete, and actionable data.

We need to improve the way platforms communicate with each other. Improving interoperability will go a long way for clinicians currently having to navigate through multiple platforms on the ambulatory, inpatient, and ancillary side to get a full medical history. Fast Healthcare Interoperability Resources (FHIR) is an IT standard describing data formats for exchanging electronic health records.

In 2020, CMS issued their Interoperability and Patient Access final rule requiring the use of FHIR by a variety of CMS-regulated payers by 2021. This rule specifically requires FHIR application programming interfaces (APIs) for patient access, provider directory, and payer-to-payer exchange. These changes now allow third-party apps to interface with the EHR to increase their functionality. A prime example includes apps that interface with sensors to check patient vitals at home and virtually enter the results in the EHR. We need to have interoperability standards in place, so developers don't need to rebuild their apps for each EHR.

At a higher level, we need to standardize and reduce payer-imposed requirements. EHRs were designed to comply with regulatory and billing mandates. However, payers vary their documentation requirements as a strategy to deny claims. CMS is now making strides in changing its requirements to make charting easier. We should require private payers to follow in CMS' footsteps to develop a uniform set of documentation standards.

Finally, we should apply design thinking to put the user at the forefront. With this in mind, vendors need to involve clinicians in the design and implementation of systems to ensure that we address user needs. After all, clinicians are the ones who interact directly with patients and understand what type of information is being requested by all parties.

By improving workflows and having the right people do the work, we can improve the wellbeing of the team providing care. By enhancing EHR interoperability and usability, we can decrease the time spent looking for information and charting. Last, by reducing payer-imposed documentation requirements, health care professionals can spend more time talking with the patient directly, instead of typing on a computer.

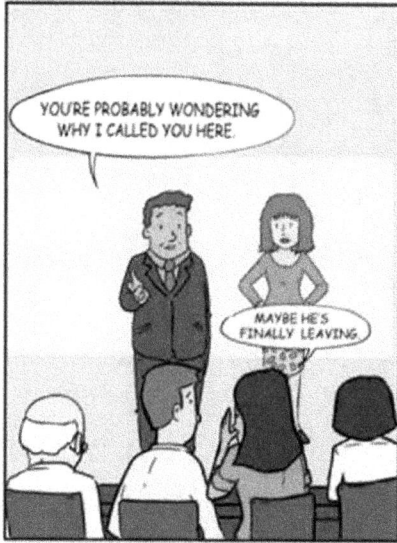

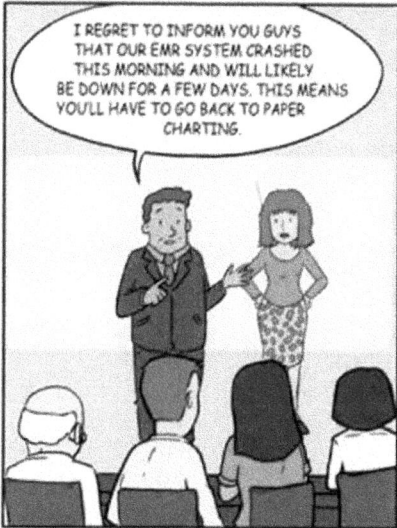

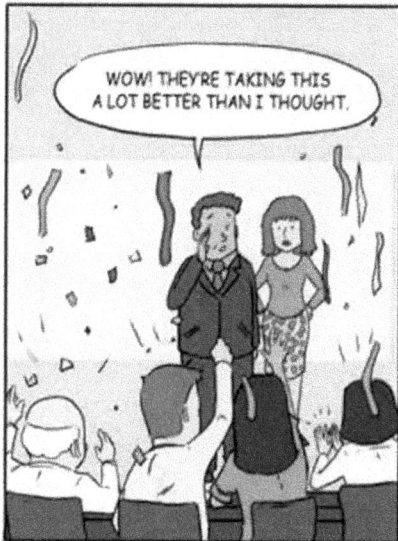

Dr. Peter Valenzuela

DOC RELATED

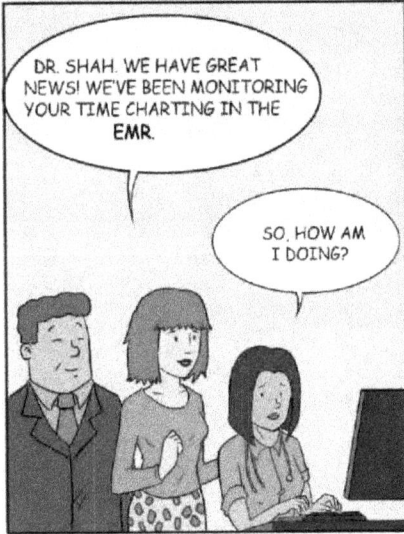

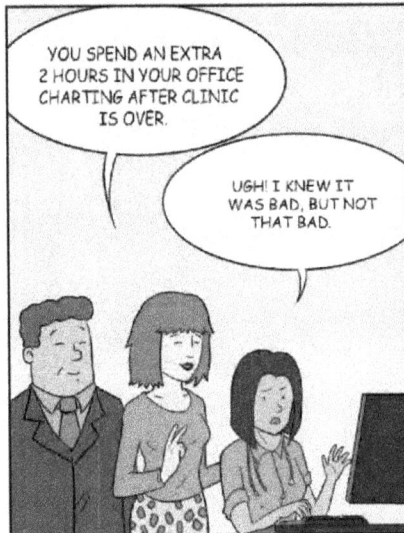

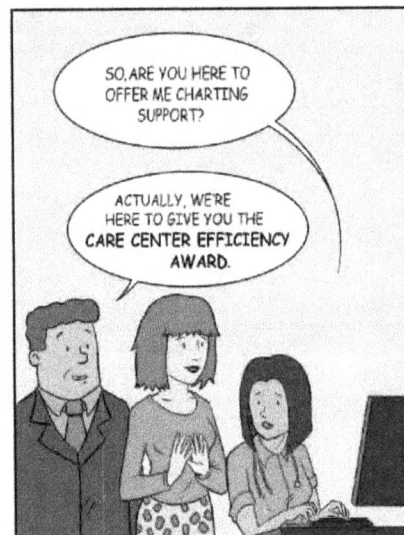

Dr. Peter Valenzuela

DOC RELATED

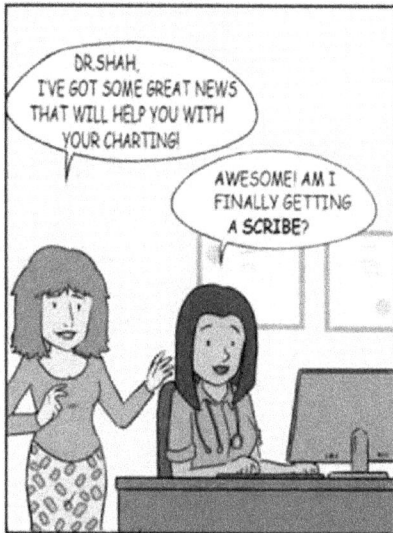

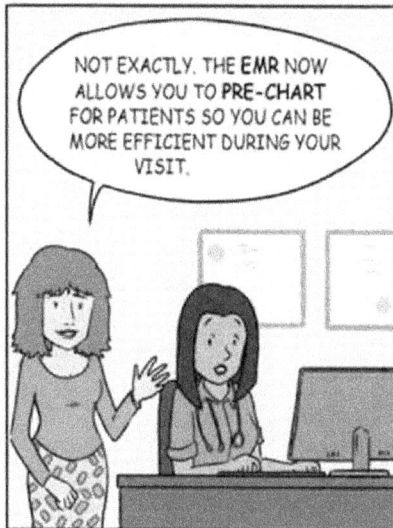

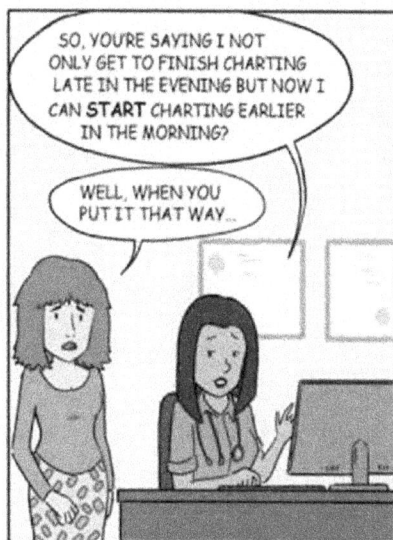

Dr. Peter Valenzuela

DOC RELATED

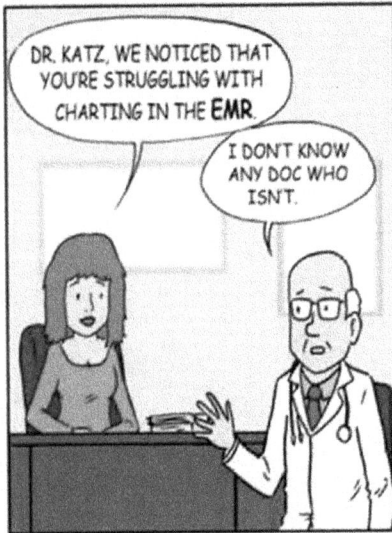

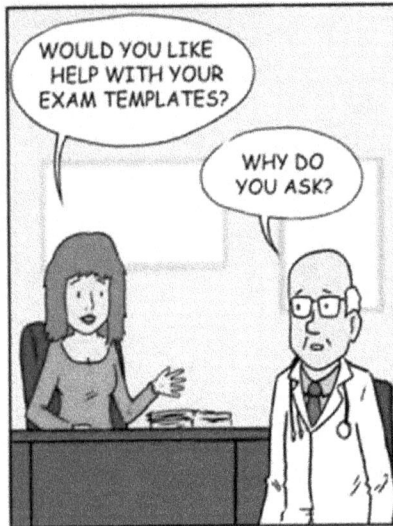

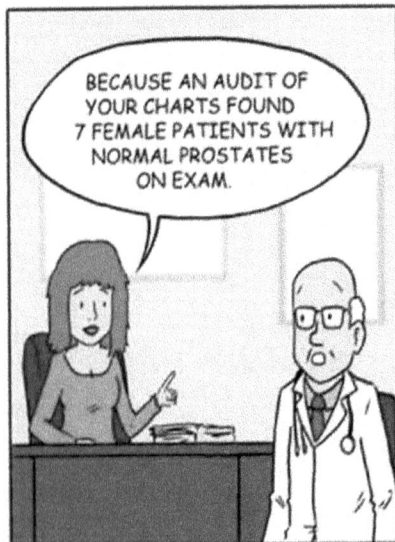

Dr. Peter Valenzuela

DOC RELATED

THIS **EMR** IS KILLING ME! I FEEL LIKE SISYPHUS WORKING AN INBASKET THAT NEVER ENDS.

WHO'S SISYPHUS?

I THINK HE WAS A DOC WHO QUIT A WHILE BACK.

OKAY, THAT MAKES SENSE TO ME NOW.

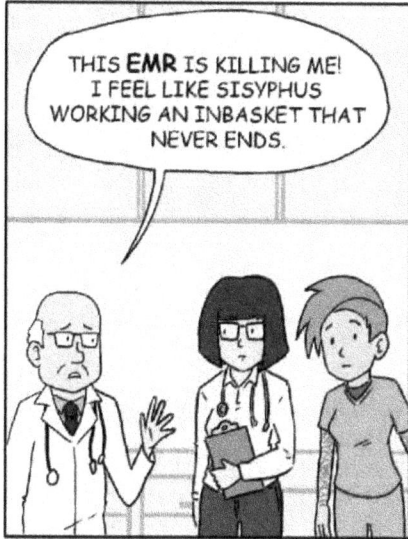

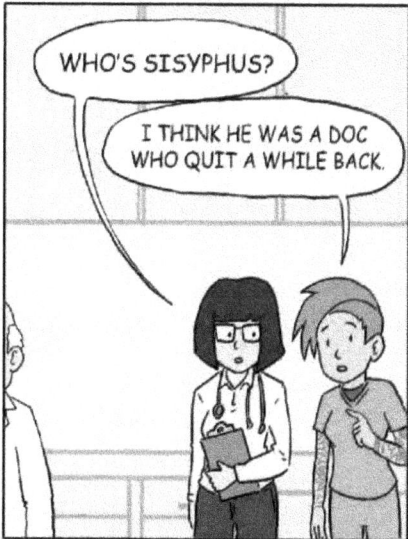

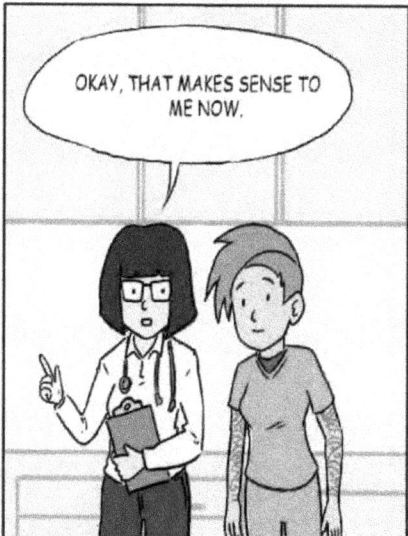

Dr .Peter Valenzuela

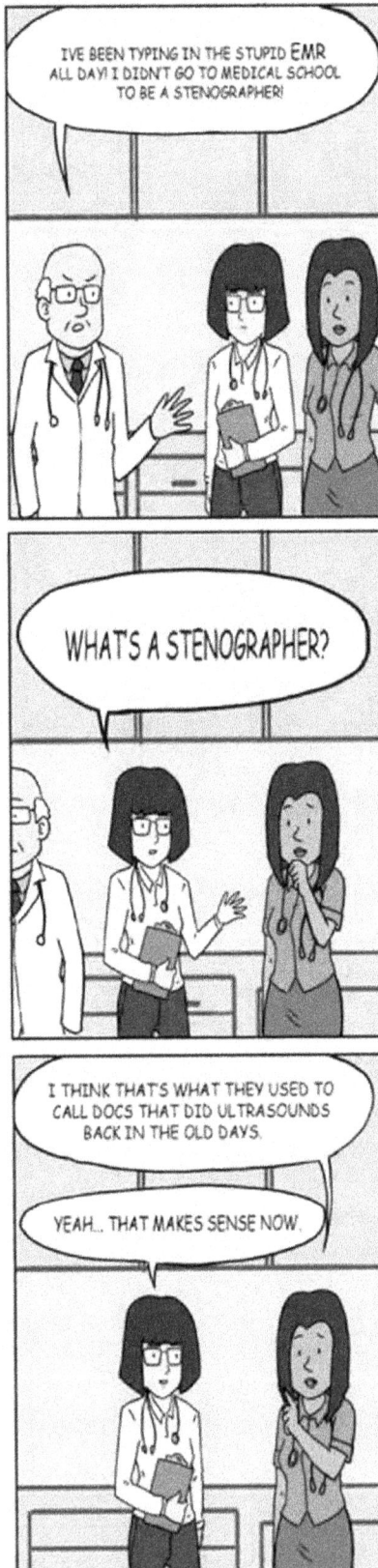

DOC RELATED

Dr. Peter Valenzuela

DOC ▬ RELATED

DONNA, SOMETHING'S WRONG WITH THE **EMR**. I CAN'T FIND THE "MEDICATION RECONCILATION" BUTTON ON THE SCREEN.

SORRY DR. KATZ, THE **EMR** SYSTEM WAS UPGRADED OVER THE WEEKEND. SOME OF THE BUTTONS WERE EITHER MOVED OR RENAMED. I THOUGHT YOU KNEW?

WHY DOES EVERY **EMR** SYSTEM UPGRADE SEEM LIKE A **DOWNGRADE** FOR DOCS?

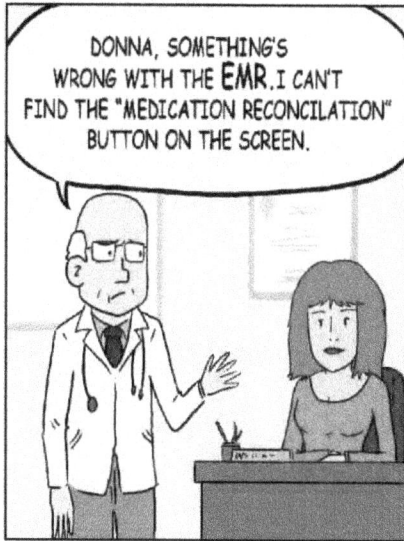

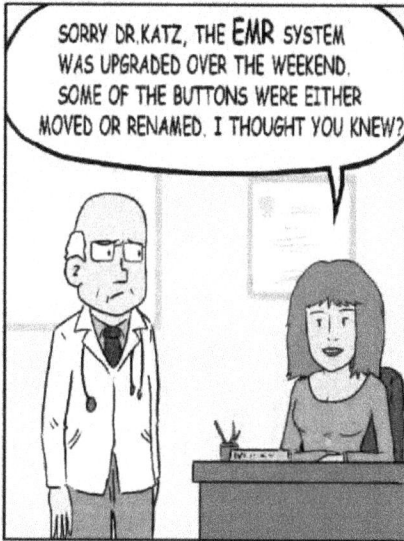

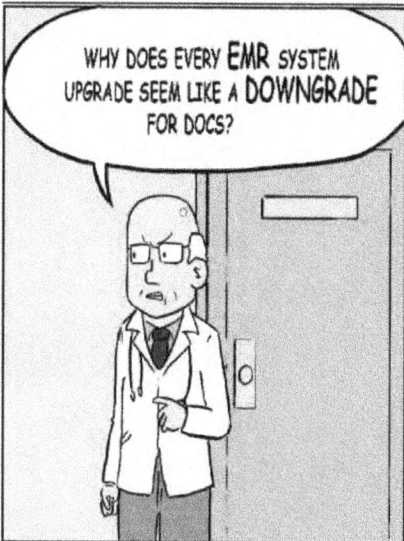

Dr. Peter Valenzuela

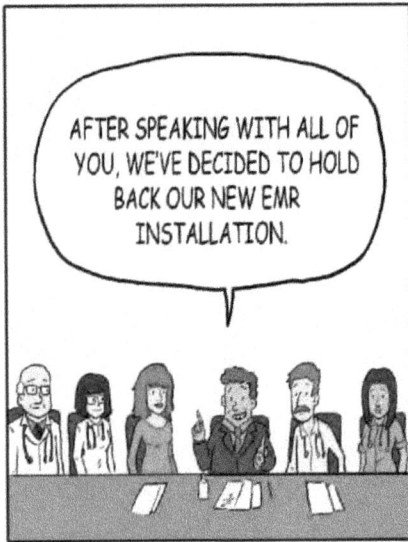

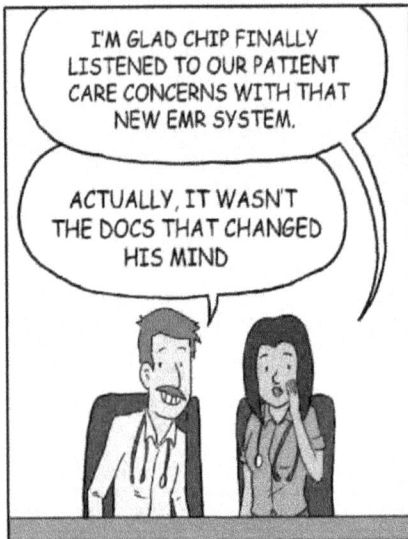

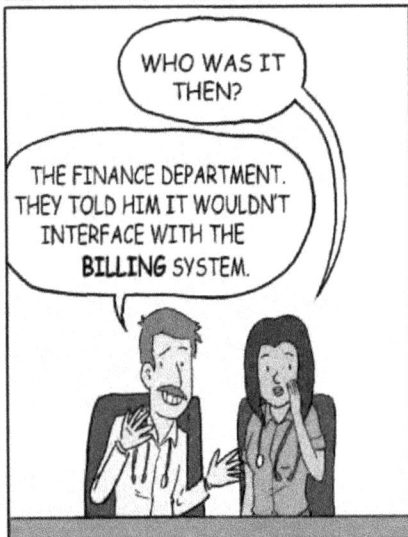

Dr. Peter Valenzuela

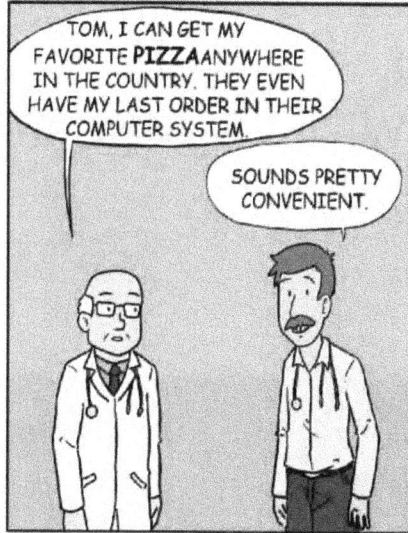

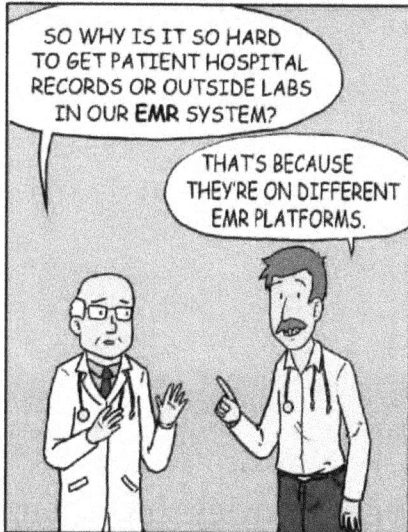

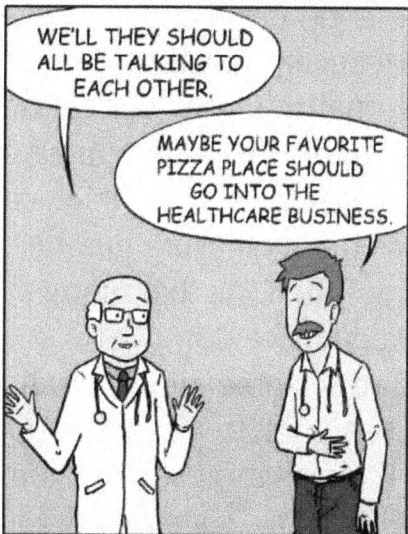

Chapter 10
Quality Metrics: Let's Change What We Measure

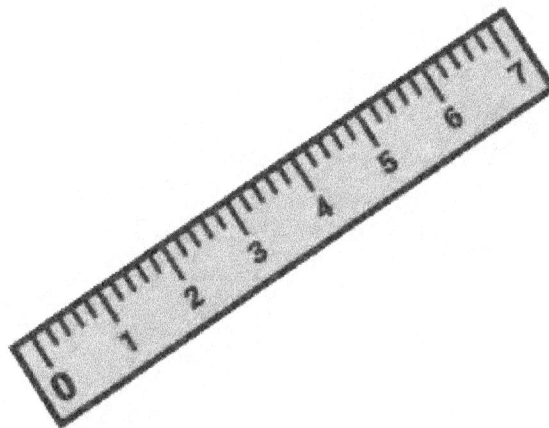

A few years ago, I sat in a quality meeting reviewing our groups' performance measures. Our presenter said, "I have good news and bad news. The good news is our quality metric for cervical cancer screening is at the 90th percentile in the nation. The bad news is our quality metric for cervical cancer *over-screening* is terrible." (Over-screening occurs when intervals between screenings are shorter than recommended guidelines.) Physicians are pressured to provide more screening tests to address the increasing number of quality metric requirements but penalized if done too often. At that moment, I thought to myself, we're damned if we do and damned if we don't.

Almost everything you read nowadays includes some blurb on how much we spend on healthcare in the U.S. and how poorly we compare to other countries. Below are a few bullets from the Organisation for Economic Co-operation (OECD) that include the U.S., Australia, Canada, France, Germany, the Netherlands, New Zealand, Norway, Sweden, Switzerland, and the United Kingdom.

- The U.S. spends more on health care as a share of the economy — nearly twice as much as the average OECD country — yet has the lowest life expectancy and highest suicide rates among the 11 nations.
- The U.S. has the highest chronic disease burden and an obesity rate that is two times higher than the OECD average.
- Compared to peer nations, the U.S. has among the highest number of hospitalizations from preventable causes and the highest rate of avoidable deaths.

The high cost of health care led the CMS and private insurers to pressure health care providers to lower expenditures and improve outcomes. They do this by developing pay-for-performance frameworks using quality metrics like cervical cancer screening rates and testing hemoglobin A1c levels (blood sugar averages) in diabetes. Also, public report cards and rankings from non-profit organizations like the Joint Commission and Leapfrog — along with for-profit organizations like Healthgrades and U.S. News & World Report — have forced health care providers to worry about their reputation for quality and safety.

Done well, measuring quality can be a good thing. However, we've gone a bit overboard. The CMS has approximately 1,700 measures for providers within different practice settings. Combine that with over 80 Healthcare Effectiveness Data and Information Set (HEDIS) measures used to score health insurance plans along with another 57 measures the Joint Commission uses to gauge the quality of inpatient care for hospitals, and you get an unsurmountable number of metrics.

To complicate matters, the metrics are not universal across all entities. For example, CMS's 2018 Shared Savings Program metric for poor diabetes control was a hemoglobin A1c level at or above 8 percent, but most health plans used the HEDIS standard of at or above 9 percent. The same applies to blood pressure control in elderly patients. Depending on the organization, systolic blood pressure targets for patients over sixty-five range from less than 130 mm Hg to less than 150 mm Hg. In fact, a study of twenty-three health insurers found they used 546 quality measures, and few of them matched across all insurers.

Reporting and collecting data is time-consuming and cumbersome. Even though most physicians use electronic health records, EHRs automate only a portion of quality metrics. This forces physicians and staff to manually track measure specifications, collect and enter data, and transmit the data.

One study of four common specialties (general internists, family physicians, cardiologists, and orthopedists) showed that physicians and staff spent 15.1 hours per physician per week dealing with quality measures, with 2.6 of those hours per week by the physicians. Time spent by physicians and staff translates to an average cost to a practice of $40,069 per physician per year. Primary care practices spent $50,468, compared to $34,924 for cardiology practices and $31,471 for orthopedics practices. They based this estimate on actual cost without considering the opportunity cost of what doctors and other personnel might have done with the time they spent capturing and inputting data.

Although the metrics may be well-intended, they don't always follow the real world of practicing medicine. Let's take the asthma medication ratio (AMR) metric. We categorize medications for asthma into long-term "controller" (steroid) medications used to maintain control of persistent asthma and short-term "rescue" (albuterol) medications used to treat acute symptoms. Appropriate ratios for these medications might prevent asthma-related hospitalizations, emergency room visits, missed work, and school days. The goal is not to overly prescribe rescue inhalers alone.

Here's the problem, patients rarely have only ONE rescue inhaler. Some of my best-controlled asthmatics—who will never need controller medication —keep a rescue inhaler at home, in the car, at school, and at work. This metric would penalize me for not prescribing a controller inhaler.

Even if appropriately prescribing the correct ratio of rescue and controller medications, they base this metric on claims data, which is what the insurance paid. As a physician, if I prescribe a patient one rescue inhaler and one controller to use each month, the claims data may show that within six months, the patient filled the rescue medication 6 times and the controller medication only twice. This makes the AMR equal to 0.25 (2 controllers divided by 2 controllers plus 6 rescue inhalers). Despite my best efforts, I miss the quality target.

The same holds true when doctors order labs or screening tests on patients who do not follow through with the orders. If the metric being tracked by the patient's insurer is claim-based, doctors will not receive credit for their efforts. Physicians are inherently competitive and hate to score lower than their colleagues in any category, especially quality. In addition, more and more physicians are being financially incentivized to achieve quality goals, so missing targets negatively affect their income.

Are We Measuring What Matters?

With quality metrics, we only measure things we can track, not necessarily what matters to the physicians treating patients. Most of the metrics tracked, such as annual screening tests, are primary care focused. Many are SMART metrics — specific, measurable, achievable, relevant, and timely. Unfortunately, finding SMART metrics for each specialty can be challenging. This can leave some specialists tracking metrics with minimal significance to the care they provide.

Another challenge with tracking quality metrics is assessing whether they truly affect overall health. Despite being a $3.6 trillion annual expense, health care delivery drives only 10-20 percent of health outcomes. Behavioral and social determinants of health — like having a job, eating right, not over-consuming alcohol, avoiding drugs, and hazardous behavior — play a much bigger role in overall health and longevity. However, they are not actively tracked.

Unintended Consequences

Although quality metrics are meant to improve patient care, reporting them can lead to negative behavior. In 2012, Medicare began financially penalizing acute care hospitals for the number of patients who return for a second stay within a month. Since implementing this penalty, hospital readmissions have declined, which many attribute to the success of performance metrics. However, when you look behind the exam curtain, many of the patients who returned to the hospital were admitted on "observation status." Patients on observation can stay in the hospital for 1-2 days without being counted as full admissions. Between 2006 and 2013, observation stays for Medicare patients increased by 96 percent. Essentially, half of the reduction in readmissions was actually because patients who had returned to the hospital were treated as outpatients.

It's just as easy to game quality metrics on the ambulatory side. The HEDIS measure for "avoidance of antibiotic treatment in adults with acute bronchitis" is determined by whether physicians prescribed antibiotics for seven ICD-10 diagnosis codes showing acute bronchitis (J20.3, J20.4, J20.5, J20.6, J20.7, J20.8, and J20.9). The way physicians get around this is by prescribing antibiotics using different ICD-10 codes that describe bronchitis symptoms, like cough (R05). Similar concepts apply to two other HEDIS metrics related to avoiding antibiotic prescribing for upper respiratory infections and ear infections.

Quality metrics and report cards can also lead to "cherry-picking" patients more likely to follow clinical recommendations. Because physicians value their reputation, they may be "risk averse" and avoid operating on patients with multiple chronic conditions who might be high-risk. Many of those patients will never undergo needed treatments. Physicians may refer some to other care centers who will then be responsible for the quality metrics. For example, as of 2015, Medicare penalized about three-quarters of the hospitals reporting 30-day readmission rates. Major teaching hospitals, which see more low income and sicker patients, were penalized more.

Ways to Fix Metrics

The easiest way to improve quality metric reporting is to cut down on the number of metrics. One of my biggest healthcare idols is Dr. Don Berwick. He's a pediatrician, former Administrator of the CMS, and former Chief Executive Officer of the Institute for Healthcare Improvement. Dr. Berwick believes we need to stop excessive measurement and reduce all metrics by 50%. He's not the only expert who supports this concept. A study by the National Academy of Medicine outlined key themes we should use to improve our reporting system. Below are a few of those themes:

- We should focus quality metric reporting on process improvement. We should target improvements that impact how we care for patients in the present. Most of what we measure has a 1-2-year time delay. This time delay limits the benefit of performance feedback in making improvements and changing physician behavior.
- We need to get all the entities requesting quality metrics to align and standardize their definitions. We should have one standard for each metric, not variances depending on the

accrediting organization or insurance company. By definition, we should all be following the best practice for each condition.

- We should design electronic health records to more easily collect and report metrics. Instead of putting the burden of data collection on healthcare providers, we should mandate that all certified EHRs abstract reporting data. Taking it one step further, we need to push for more interoperability, so the EHRs talk to each other. This will allow us to track metrics performed outside of individual care centers and decrease redundant testing.

- We should move away from quality metrics derived from billing and administrative systems. We should not penalize physicians and clinicians for doing the right thing, only to have the patient not follow recommendations.

Besides the recommendations above, we need to develop quality metrics that are specialty specific. All physicians should have the ability to develop quality metrics that matter to them. Choosing Wisely is an initiative of the American Board of Internal Medicine (ABIM) Foundation that promotes patient-physician conversations about unnecessary medical tests and procedures. The program launched in 2012 and includes 54 specialty societies and 17 consumer groups. Choosing Wisely asks each clinician group to create a list of practices that are overused, following these guidelines:

- Practices should be used frequently and/or carry a significant cost.
- There should be generally accepted evidence to support each recommendation.
- Each item should be within the purview and control of the organization's members.
- The process should be thoroughly documented and publicly available upon request.

Choosing Wisely now has over 550 recommendations developed by clinicians for clinicians. A few examples include not performing MRIs of the peripheral joints to routinely monitor inflammatory arthritis in rheumatology and avoiding opioids for migraines, except as a last resort in neurology.

In addition, we need to incorporate metrics that matter to patients and impact overall health. The greatest way is by addressing social determinants, which make up 80-90% of a person's overall health. Examples include opportunities and resources in homes, neighborhoods, and communities, along with the quality of our schooling, the safety of our workplaces, and the cleanliness of our water, food, and air. By shifting the roughly $15 billion physicians spend reporting metrics annually to target social determinants, we can institute programs that matter.

Last, there are over 318,000 health apps available today, with over 200 apps being added each day. We should require EHR vendors to allow third-party technologies to help clinicians better understand patient behavior. These technologies will also help patients take control of their overall health and well-being.

DOC RELATED

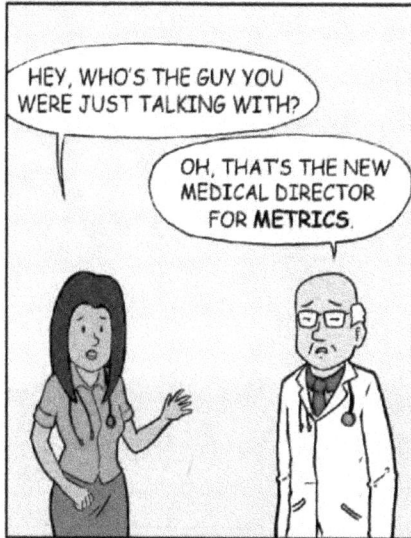

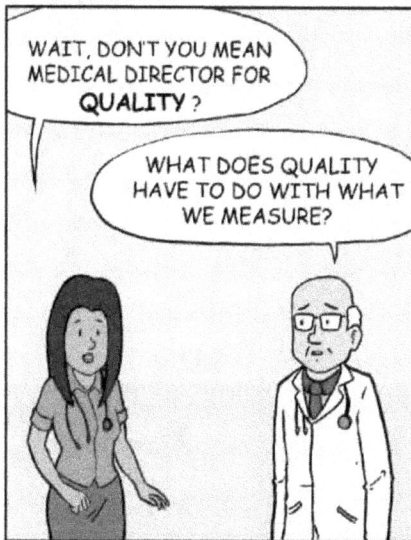

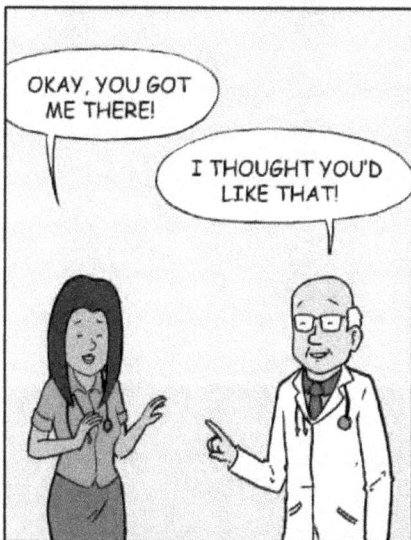

Dr. Peter Valenzuela

DOC-RELATED

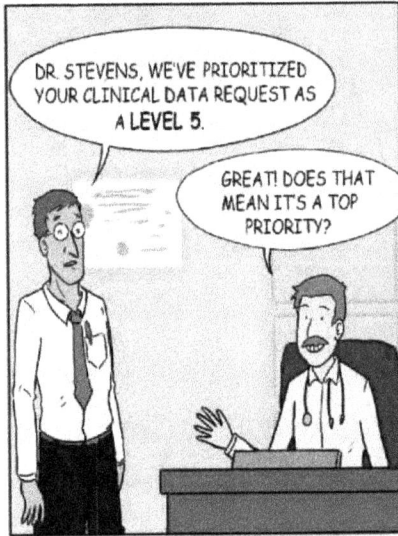

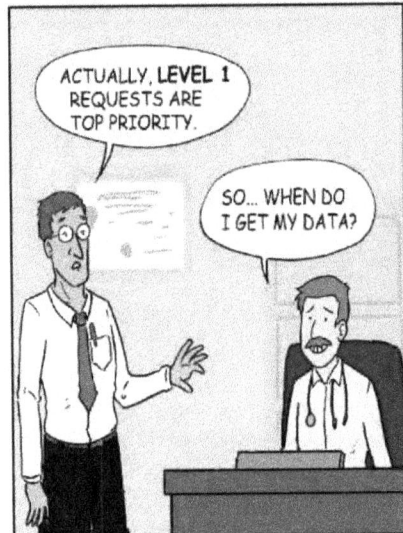

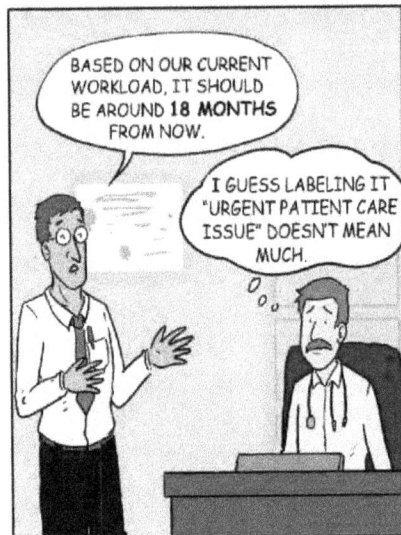

Dr. Peter Valenzuela

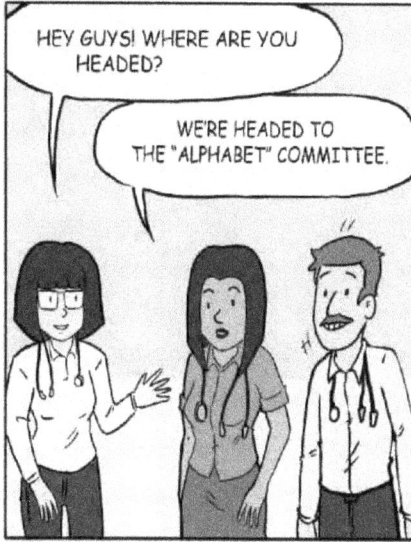

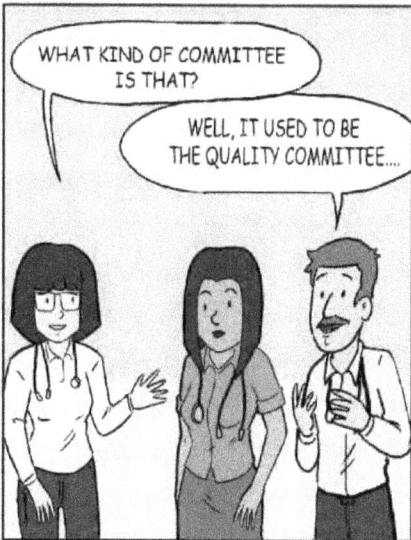

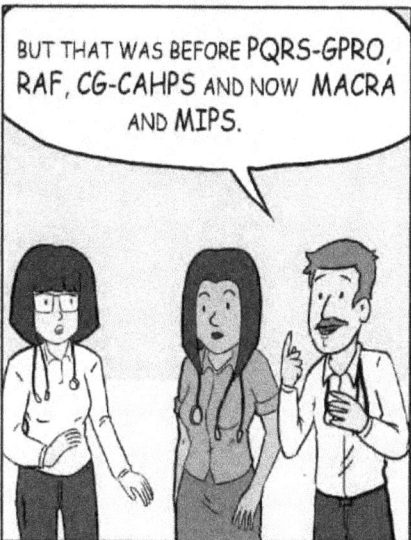

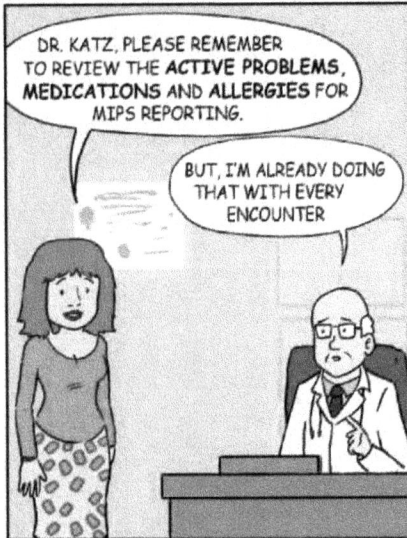

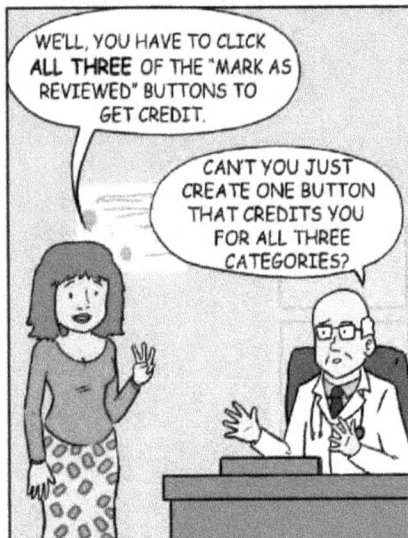

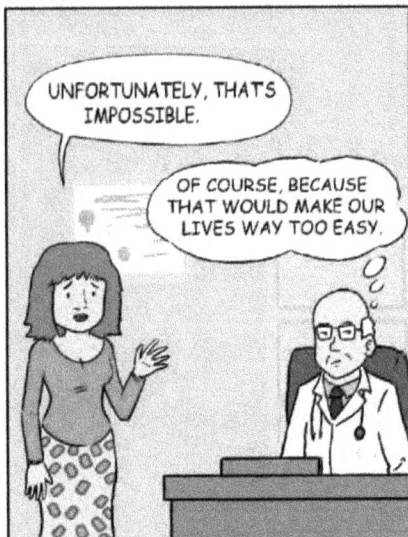

DOC-RELATED

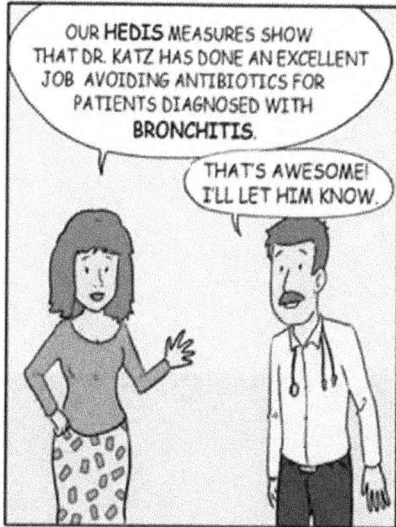

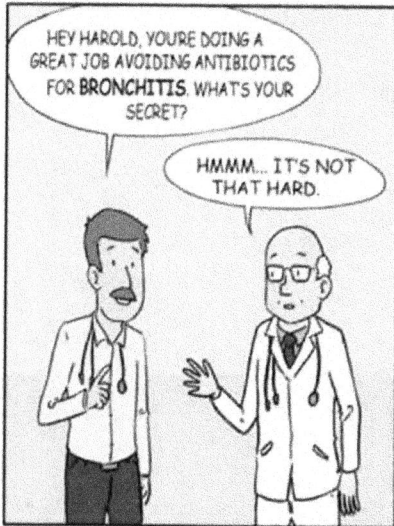

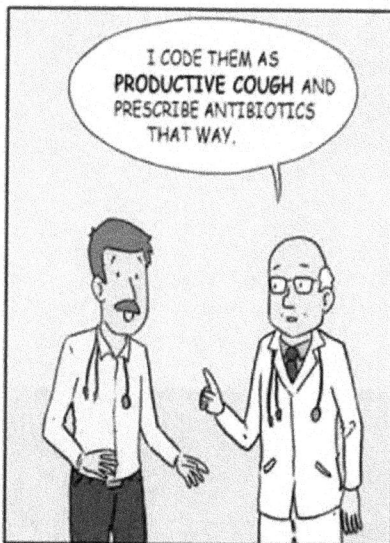

Dr. Peter Valenzuela

DOC-RELATED

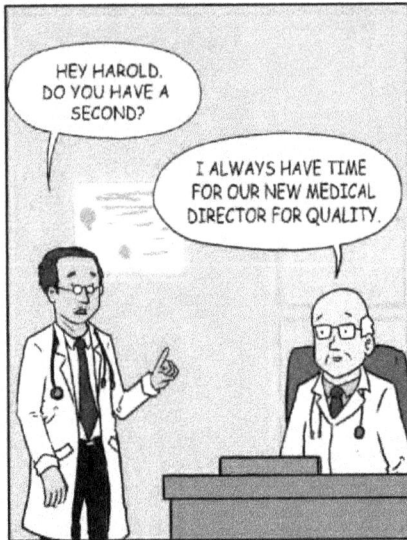

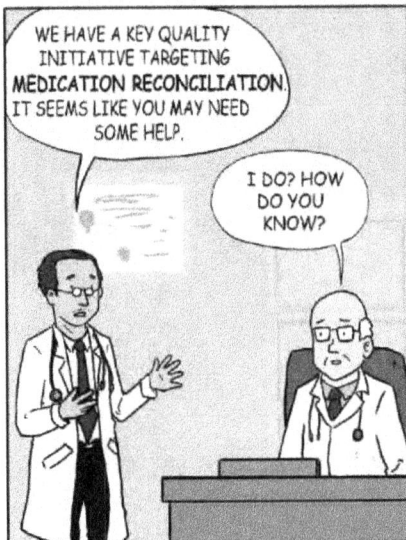

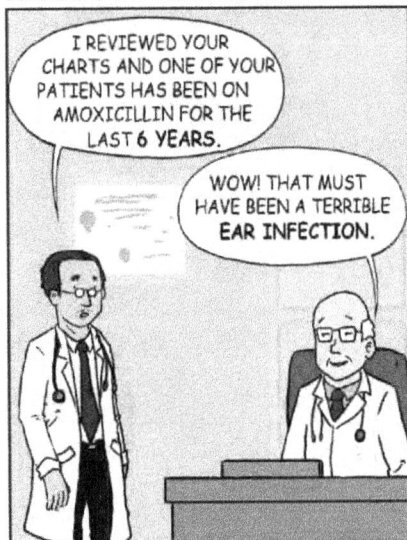

Dr. Peter Valenzuela

Chapter 11
Malpractice: The Best Offense Is a Good Defense

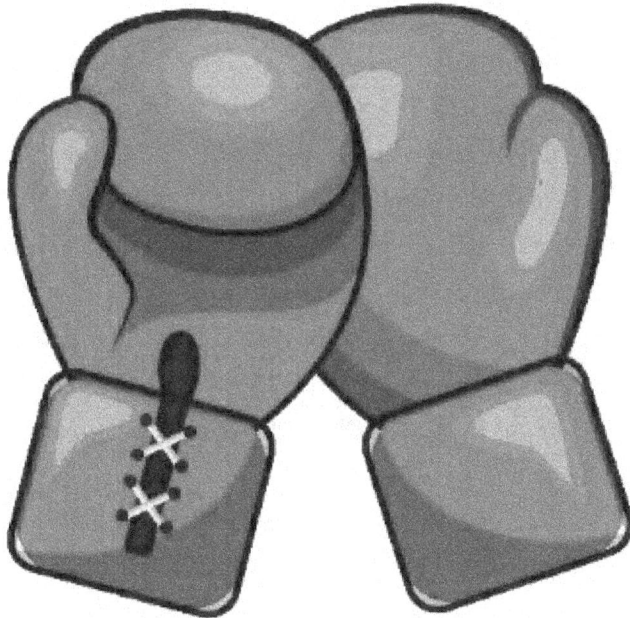

In the first section of this book, we covered how patient surveys have changed the way we care for patients and ways that leadership and communication impact provider engagement and staff satisfaction. We also touched on the need to have adequate staff working at the top of their licensure to improve operations.

Section two covered how health care providers are paid, including the impact of coding and prior authorizations on payments. This section also covered how physicians' work is measured. Section three has focused on electronic health records and the time dedicated to charting. It's also covered quality metrics and the need to find a better way to influence patient outcomes. The last chapter in this section addresses the icing on the bureaucratic cake—how fear of malpractice lawsuits has affected patient care.

Two years after starting my practice as a rural physician in West Texas, the family of a patient I never met sued me. The patient was a female in her twenties, brought to the emergency room from the county jail after complaining of fatigue and depressed moods. Like many small hospitals in the early 2000s, a physician assistant (PA) staffed our emergency room. The (PA) evaluated the patient and diagnosed her with depression. He prescribed an anti-depressant and placed her on suicide precautions when he discharged her back to the county jail. He also recommended she be seen by a behavioral health specialist within the next 1-2 weeks. Six months later, she committed suicide after being transferred to a women's prison.

Her mother was so grief-stricken that she hired a malpractice attorney. Her attorney filed a "shotgun" lawsuit, naming anyone who had anything to do with her daughter's visit to the emergency room — including the hospital CEO. Attorneys file shotgun suits with the sole purpose of finding someone they could intimidate into paying a settlement just to get out of the lawsuit. They named me in the lawsuit because I was the physician on call the day the patient presented to the ER. Her encounter was so routine, the PA never even called me to discuss the case.

Over the next few months, I spent time in depositions discussing my role in the lawsuit and being interrogated about standards of care and emergency room protocols. Attorneys have a way of disorienting facts, so I began doubting myself and wondering how I could have prevented her death. It was a demoralizing experience. In the end, they dismissed the case with no fault found in any of the defendants. This frivolous lawsuit took a year to resolve but left a scar on me as a young physician just starting his career. It also had a financial toll because of the time spent away from my practice.

I'm not alone. More than a third of physicians (34 percent) have had a claim filed against them in their careers. The risk increases the longer a physician practices. Roughly half (49.2 percent) of physicians age 55 and over have been sued. Lawsuits vary by specialty. Over half of all general surgeons, OB/GYNs, and emergency medicine physicians have been sued compared to 18 percent of pediatricians and 16 percent of psychiatrists. Gender also plays a role in that female physicians are less likely to be sued than male physicians. Almost 40 percent of male physicians have been sued over the course of their careers, compared to 22.8 percent of women.

Outcomes

Based on the number of malpractice claims, you'd assume there are a lot of medical errors occurring. However, data shows that most liability claims have no merit. Sixty-five percent of claims that closed between 2016 and 2018 were dropped, dismissed, or withdrawn. Out of six percent of claims that were decided by a trial verdict, the defendant (physician) won almost 90 percent in the case. Even though most cases get dropped, getting to a resolution takes time. The average time from claim filing to close is 20 months for cases with no payment and may take three or more years for those ending with a payment.

Speaking from experience, the stress and anxiety of a malpractice case can be overwhelming while you are still trying to care for patients. Even if you win, you may end up losing. The average cost to defend a claim that eventually gets dropped or dismissed is $30,439 7, not including time away from work. Insurers may also increase malpractice insurance premiums after a lawsuit. In some states, physicians pay over $200,000 a year in insurance premiums just to practice medicine.

How Malpractice Lawsuits Impact Patients

In the same way that physicians are affected by the long legal process, patients and their families are often forced to wait years for a resolution. In the meantime, they handle the expenses of dealing with the alleged error, which is often not purely financial. If a patient has suffered harm, it may require multiple surgeries, continued therapy, and prolonged — sometimes permanent — disability. Should the court find fault in the health care provider and award an indemnity payment, the attorney is entitled to as much as 40 percent. Lawyers justify the exorbitant amount by accounting for expert medical witness fees, court filing fees, and the cost of obtaining medical records from hospitals or care centers.

Along with the cost of dealing with malpractice liability, fear of lawsuits affects how physicians care for patients. We call this defensive medicine. Estimates of the cost of defensive medicine per year vary between $46 billion and $78 billion dollars. Some sources estimate it to be as high as $300 billion dollars. There are two types of defensive medicine—positive and negative. Positive defensive medicine is ordering more tests or procedures to reduce malpractice liability. It's done to assure patients that all avenues have been investigated and checked off. Sixty percent of physicians acknowledge ordering tests or consultations simply to avoid the appearance of malpractice.

Negative defensive medicine is avoiding patients who are high-risk or performing high-risk procedures. It can also be avoiding practicing in certain geographies. Studies show physicians may avoid inner cities because of sicker populations, higher rates of noncompliance and missed appointments, limited ability to truly affect social determinants of health, and perceptions that malpractice suits are more likely to occur in these areas. This results in those patients not receiving care that they truly need.

Negative defensive medicine is seen in obstetricians, who are among the highest specialties involved in lawsuits. A 2015 survey from the American College of Obstetricians and Gynecologists (ACOG) found that 49.7 percent have altered their practices, including accepting less high-risk patients, increasing cesarean births, and decreasing the overall number of deliveries. A 2010 New Physician Workforce Study in Illinois found that 49 percent of new physicians planned to move to a different state because of the medical liability environment , resulting in less access to care for patients.

Ways to Fix Malpractice

As clinicians, we ground our ethical obligations in the principles of autonomy, beneficence, and non-maleficence and the virtues of compassion, courage, and honesty. I'm not advocating that all malpractice suits are without merit. If we commit mistakes beyond the standard of care or egregiously, the patient should be allowed some level of remuneration. However, we should look at how we address most cases that end up being dismissed, dropped, or withdrawn.

One of the first ways to do this is to permit physicians to acknowledge their mistakes without fear of litigation. We need to learn from mistakes to improve processes and patient care. State apology laws are not written in ways that foster open and honest communication between the physician and the injured party. Twenty-five states have "sympathy only" laws. This type of law prevents an expression of sympathy (e.g., "I'm sorry") from being entered into evidence as proof of malpractice.

Recently, the Agency for Healthcare Research and Quality (AHRQ) developed the Communication for Optimal Resolution (CANDOR) toolkit to address this issue. The CANDOR process uses a patient-centered approach to early disclosure of adverse events. This method targets an amicable and fair resolution for the patient, family, and health care providers involved. This helps to foster open communication between health care providers and patients after unanticipated health outcomes.

Being sued is extremely stressful. Physicians should have peer support to guide them through the process. Most physicians prefer support from colleagues rather than mental health practitioners during stressful times and talking with colleagues after medical errors have been shown to improve physician resilience. Peer supporters can also facilitate connections with mental health services by de-stigmatizing these services and facilitating access to them.

To truly affect change, we should have national legislation that limits non-economic damages in liability cases. Noneconomic damages mean damages arising from pain, suffering, inconvenience, physical impairment, mental anguish, emotional pain, and suffering. Currently, twenty-six states cap non-economic damages in medical malpractice claims, while six have "total caps" that limit both economic and non-economic compensation.

We should also have legislation that puts a cap on attorney fees and payments. If a patient is awarded money for damages, we should limit their attorney to a contingency fee that does not exceed more than a certain percentage of the total reward. As I write this book, the California health care community is fighting the "Fairness for Injured Patients Act" that we will vote on in 2022. This act will eliminate the cap on non-economic damages and the cap on attorney's fees in medical malpractice cases, allowing lawyers to take up to 50% of a patient's jury award in malpractice cases. This ballot measure is being led by a single trial lawyer looking to increase lawyers' share of medical malpractice awards.

Having a safe environment for physicians to admit and learn from negative outcomes is the first step. Supporting them in the process is the second. Establishing legislation to limit non-economic damages is the third. Capping attorney fees is the fourth. These types of reform will also increase physicians in underserved areas, decrease spending on unnecessary procedures, lower health insurance premiums, and reduce Medicaid spending.

DOC RELATED

Panel 1:
HEY TOM, I JUST SAW A PATIENT WHO THOUGHT SHE HAD EVERY CONDITION KNOWN TO MEDICINE.

YEAH, I'VE HAD A FEW OF THOSE BEFORE.

Panel 2:
I ENDED UP ORDERING ALL KINDS OF UNNECESSARY LABS AND IMAGING STUDIES FOR HER.

WHAT MADE YOU DO THAT?

Panel 3:
SHE'S A **LAWYER.**

YEP. I'VE **DEFINITELY** HAD A FEW OF THOSE BEFORE.

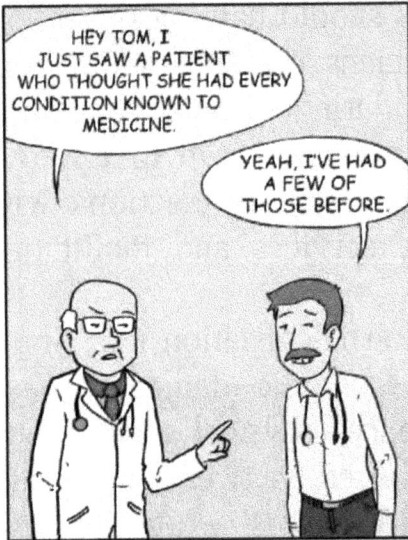

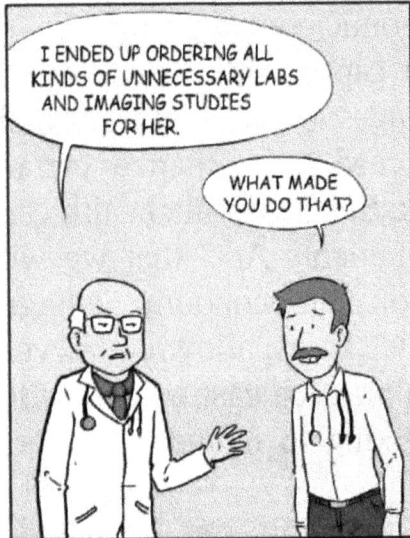

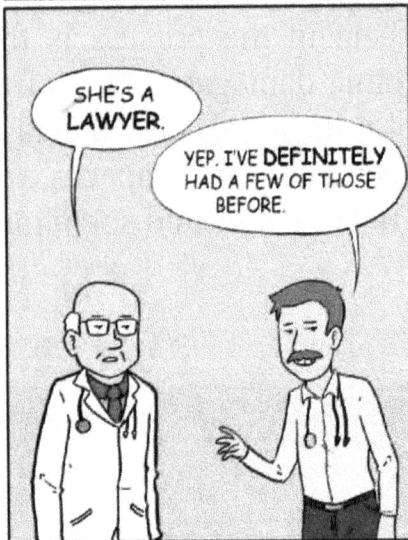

Dr. Peter Valenzuela

DOC RELATED

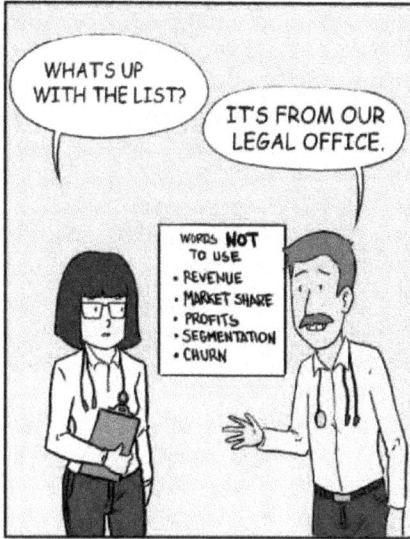

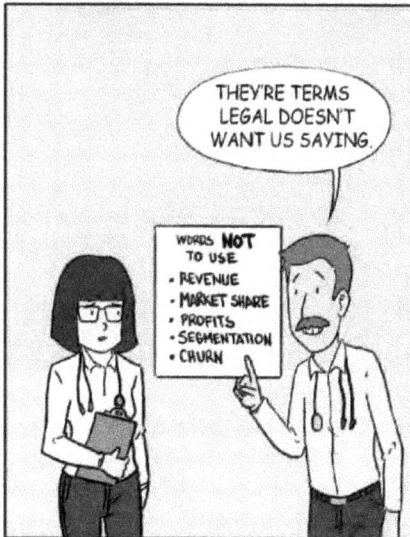

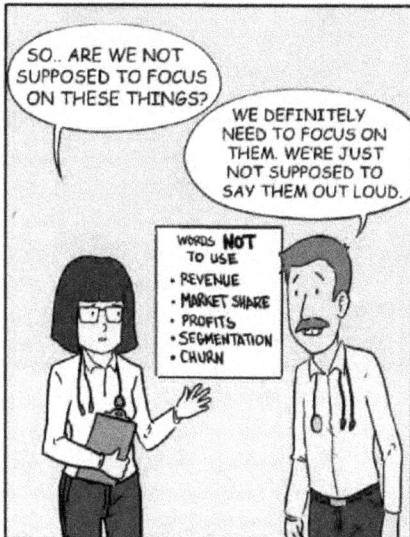

Dr. Peter Valenzuela

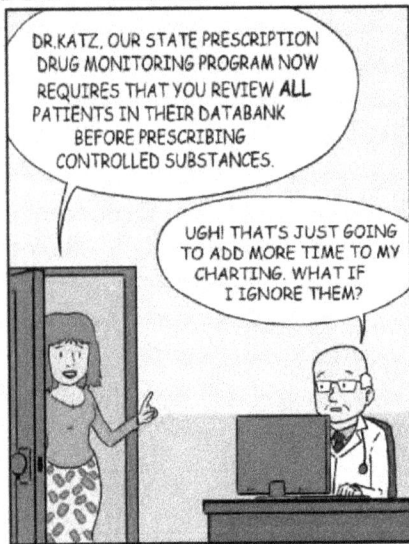

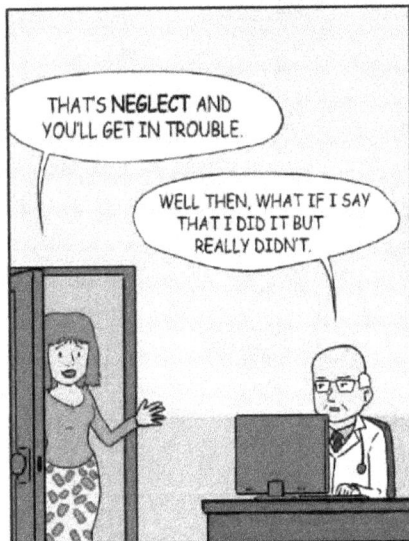

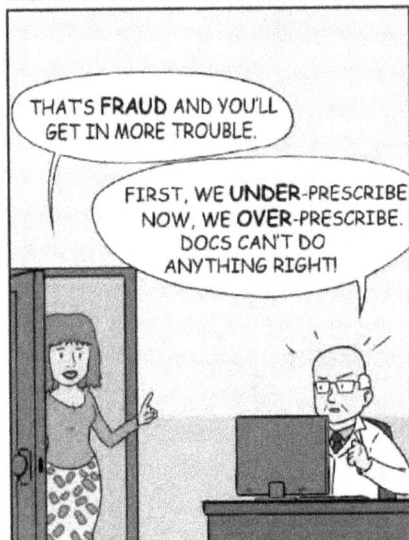

DOC—RELATED

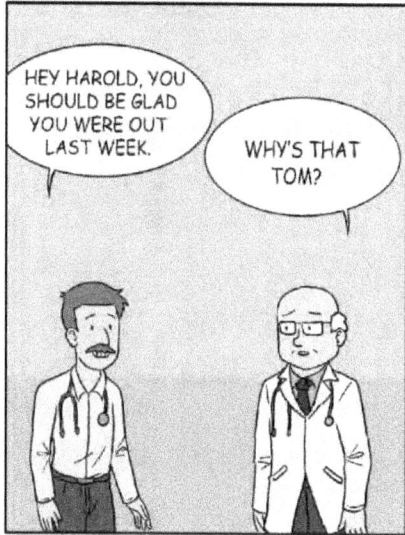

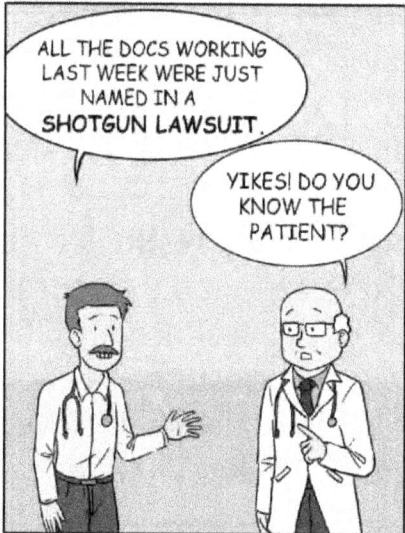

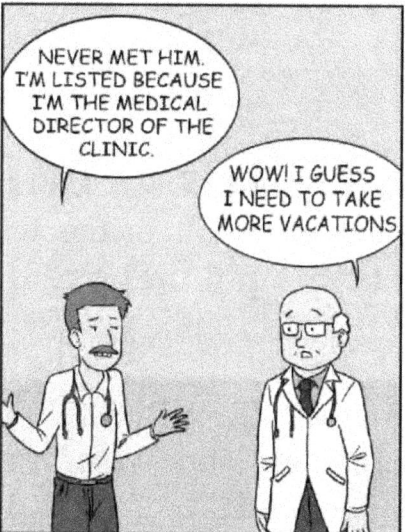

Dr .Peter Valenzuela

Notes and References

Introduction

1. **over 16 million people in the industry:** Derek Thompson. "Healthcare Just Became the U.S.'s Largest Employer," *The Atlantic*, January 9, 2018, https://www.theatlantic.com/business/archive/2018/01/healthcare-america-jobs/550079/

2. **Nearly 70% of U.S. physicians are employed by hospitals or corporate entities:** "COVID-19's Impact on Acquisitions of Physician Practices and Physician Employment 2019-2020," Avaleri Health, Report from the Physician Advocacy Institute, June 2021.

3. **consider the impact of strategic decisions on the resilience and well-being of those affected:** "Human Experience at the Forefront: Elevating Resilience, Well-being, and Joy in Healthcare," 2016 Research Report, Experience Innovation Network, Part of Vocera.

4. **Comedians have become the truth tellers:** Malcolm Gladwell, "The Satire Paradox," Revisionist History Podcast, https://www.pushkin.fm/episode/the-satire-paradox/

Chapter 1: Meet the Crew

5. **Baby boomers currently comprise 25% of the U.S. workforce:** Richard Fry, "Millennials are the largest generation in the U.S. labor force," Pew Research Center, April 11, 2018, https://www.pewresearch.org/fact-tank/2018/04/11/millennials-largest-generation-us-labor-force/

6. **They comprise 33% of the labor force in the U.S.:** Richard Fry, "Millennials are the largest generation in the U.S. labor force," Pew Research Center, April 11, 2018, https://www.pewresearch.org/fact-tank/2018/04/11/millennials-

largest-generation-us-labor-force/

7. **They comprise 35% of the U.S. Workforce and approximately 15% still live at home with their parents:** Richard Fry, "Millennials are the largest generation in the U.S. labor force," Pew Research Center, April 11, 2018, https://www.pewresearch.org/fact-tank/2018/04/11/millennials-largest-generation-us-labor-force/

8. **Most Interesting Man in the World from Dos Equis commercials:** Wikipedia, The Most Interesting Man in the World, https://en.wikipedia.org/wiki/The_Most_Interesting_Man_in_the_W

9. **Generation Z — those born between 1995-2015:** Michael Dimock, "Defining generations: Where Millennials end and Generation Z begins," Pew Research Center, January 17, 2019, https://www.pewresearch.org/fact-tank/2019/01/17/where-millennials-end-and-generation-z-begins/

Chapter 2: The Quest for Positive Reviews

10. **Vernon and Nelle:** Not actual names.

11. **older, sicker patients who generate higher health care costs rate their providers better** : R C Ford, S A Bach, M D Fottler, "Methods for Measuring Patient Satisfaction in Health Care Organizations. Ford," Health Care Management Review, Spring 1997. https://pubmed.ncbi.nlm.nih.gov/9143904/

12. **demands are different for new physicians with whom they haven't established a relationship:** R C Ford, S A Bach, M D Fottler, "Methods for Measuring Patient Satisfaction in Health Care Organizations. Ford," Health Care Management Review, Spring 1997. https://pubmed.ncbi.nlm.nih.gov/9143904/

13. **CG-CAHPs raw percentage score of 85:** "2019 Adult 6-Month Survey 3.0 with/without PCMH items Percentiles," Agency for Healthcare Research and Quality CAHP Surveys and Tools to Advance Patient-Centered Care, 2019, Accessed July 7, 2021, https://cahpsdatabase.ahrq.gov/CAHPSIDB/CG/Percentile.aspx

14. **can give different satisfaction ratings because of their different expectations:** "What Is Patient Experience?" Agency for

Healthcare Quality and Research, https://www.ahrq.gov/cahps/about-cahps/patient-experience/index.html

15. **Studies show that those physicians with negative online reviews:** R. Jay Widmer, MD, PhD; Matthew J. Maurer, MS; Veena R. Nayar, MBA;Lee A. Aase, MA; John T. Wald, MD; Amy L. Kotsenas, MD; Farris K. Timimi, MD;Charles M. Harper, MD; and Sandhya Pruthi, MD, "Online Physician Reviews Do Not Reflect Patient Satisfaction Survey Responses," Mayo Clin Proc., April 2018.

16. **28 percent said the scores made them consider quitting:** A Zagierska, D Rabago, MM Miller MM, "Impact of patient satisfaction ratings on physicians and clinical care. Patient Prefer Adherence," 2014

17. **Google search for "patient satisfaction" reveals 164 MILLION results:** Google search on June 20, 2021.

18. **video has been viewed close to one million times on YouTube:** ZDoggMD, "Blank Script," YouTube. Posted January 13, 2015, https://www.youtube.com/watch?v=ay5_HgZLDoE

19. **They were 12% more likely to be admitted to the hospital and accounted for 9% more in total health care costs:** Kai Falkenberg, "Why Rating Your Doctor Is Bad For Your Health" Forbes, January 2, 2013, https://www.forbes.com/sites/kaifalkenberg/2013/01/02/why-rating-your-doctor-is-bad-for-your-health/?sh=292ca4b533c5

20. **or to raise concerns about smoking, substance abuse, or mental-health issues:** Kai Falkenberg, "Why Rating Your Doctor Is Bad For Your Health" Forbes, January 2, 2013, https://www.forbes.com/sites/kaifalkenberg/2013/01/02/why-rating-your-doctor-is-bad-for-your-health/?sh=292ca4b533c5

21. **Health Insurance Portability and Accountability Act:** "Health Insurance Portability and Accountability Act of 1996 (HIPAA)," Public Health Professonals Gateway, Centers for Disease Control and Prevention, https://www.cdc.gov/phlp/publications/topic/hipaa.html

22. **Eighty-five percent of the reasons for failure are deficiencies in the systems and process rather than the employee:** The W.

Ewards Deming Institute, https://deming.org/quotes/

Chapter 3: What Are You Saying?

23.   **trust is at an all-time low due to poor communication between administrators and physicians:** Anish Bhardwaj, "Alignment between physicians and hospital administrators: historical perspective and future directions," Hospital Practice, 2017;45(3):81-87. doi:10.1080/21548331.2017.1327302

24.   **physician engagement study that investigated the differences between physicians and hospital administrators:** Eric J. Keller, Brad Giafaglione, Howard B. Chrisman, Jeremy D. Collins, Robert L. Vogelzang, "The growing pains of physician-administration relationships in an academic medical center and the effects on physician engagement," PLOS One, February 13, 2019, https://journals.plos.org/plosone/article?id=10.1371/journal.pone.0212014

25.   **Now there's a centralized scheduling system:** Eric J. Keller, Brad Giafaglione, Howard B. Chrisman, Jeremy D. Collins, Robert L. Vogelzang, "The growing pains of physician-administration relationships in an academic medical center and the effects on physician engagement," PLOS One, February 13, 2019, https://journals.plos.org/plosone/article?id=10.1371/journal.pone.0212014

26.   **doctor burnout costs the U.S. health care system roughly $4.6 billion a year:** Shasha Han, MS, Tait D. Shanafelt, MD, Christine A. Sinsky, MD, Karim M. Awad, MD, Liselotte N. Dyrbye, MD, MHPE, Lynne C. Fiscus, MD, MPH, Mickey Trockel, MD, Joel Goh, PhD, "Estimating the Attributable Cost of Physician Burnout in the United States," Annals of Internal Medicine, June 4, 2019.

27.   **Dr. Tate Shanafelt's research on burnout and physician satisfaction highlights the role of leadership in health care:** Tait D. Shanafelt, MD, and John H. Noseworthy, MD, CE, "Executive Leadership and Physician Well-being: Nine Organizational Strategies to Promote Engagement and Reduce Burnout," Mayo Clinical Proceedings, January 2017.

28. **Hospital quality scores are approximately 25% higher in physician-run hospitals than in manager-run hospitals:** James K. Stoller, Amanda Goodall, Agnes Baker, "Why The Best Hospitals Are Managed by Doctors," Harvard Business Review, December 27, 2016 https://hbr.org/2016/12/why-the-best-hospitals-are-managed-by-doctors?referral=03759&cm_vc=rr_item_page.bottom.

29. **The same is true in high performing medical groups with physician-led governance structures**: Advisory Board. The High-Performance Medical Group: From Aggregations of Employed Practices to an Integrated Clinical Enterprise. 2011

30. **at physician-led groups, physicians tend to be more satisfied with their employer:** Bain and Company Report, "Front Line of Healthcare Report 2017: Why involving doctors can help improve US healthcare," https://www.bain.com/insights/front-line-of-healthcare-report-2017/

31. **Dr. Toby Cosgrove, past CEO of Cleveland Clinic, responded without hesitation, "credibility... peer-to-peer credibility.":** James K. Stoller, Amanda Goodall, Agnes Baker, "Why The Best Hospitals Are Managed by Doctors," Harvard Business Review, December 27, 2016 https://hbr.org/2016/12/why-the-best-hospitals-are-managed-by-doctors?referral=03759&cm_vc=rr_item_page.bottom.

32. **What happens if we invest in the developing our people and they leave?** Peter Baeklund, www.peterbaeklund.com

33. **Mayo Clinic established this structure over 100 years ago:** D Cortese, RK Smoldt, "5 success factors for physician-administrator partnerships." MGMA Insight, 2019. https://www.mgma.com/resources/business-strategy/5-success-factors-for-physician-administrator-part

34. **identify three concepts of successful corporations, including leadership, accountability, and organizational structure:** Brian Dive, "The Accountable Leader: Developing Effective Leadership Through Managerial Accountability," Kogan Page Publishing, 2008.

35. **One of my favorite — although somewhat heretical books**: Gary Hamel, "First, Let's Fire All the Managers," Harvard Business

Review, December 2011

36.   **If you're not in the jungle, you're not going to know the tiger**: Tom Kelly, "The Art of Innovation: Lessons in Creativity from IDEO, America's Leading Design Firm" Random House, New York, 2001.

37.   **can provide them a deeper understanding of these decisions on patients, clinicians, and the clinical workplace:** Paul DeChant, MD, MBA, "Building Bridges Between Practicing Physicians and Administrators," AMA STEPSforward, 2021. https://edhub.ama-assn.org/steps-forward/module/2780305?widget=personalizedcontent&previousarticle=2702556

38.   **ITW is a $14 billion company that manufactures a wide range of products:** Josh Linkner, "Disciplined Dreaming," Jossey-Bass Publishing, San Francisco, 2011.

Chapter 4: Do You Have What You Need?

39.   **vacancy rates for nurses runt at 17%** AMN Healthcare, "Clinical Workforce Survey," 2013, https://www.amnhealthcare.com/uploadedFiles/MainSite/Content/H

40.   **better performing practices reported almost 9% greater medical total operating cost per full-time-equivalent (FTE) physician:** "MGMA Better Performers Data Report: Performance and Practices of Successful Medical Groups, 2020."

41.   **Sutter Gould Medical Group**: process based on site visit and discussions with Chief Medical Officer Dr. Steve Mitnick and Chief Operating Officer Katherine Manuel in 2016.

Chapter 5: Will This Be Covered?

42.   **There are over 900 health insurance companies offering medical coverage in the U.S.:** Sterling Price, "Largest Health Insurance Companies of 2021," Value Penguin, Updated May 24, 2021. https://www.valuepenguin.com/largest-health-insurance-companies

43.   **biggest provider of insurance in the U.S. caring for**

approximately 43% of the population: "U.S. Health Care Coverage and Spending," Congressional Research Service, Updated January 26, 2021, https://fas.org/sgp/crs/misc/IF10830.pdf

44. **who control more than 44% of the market:** Sterling Price, "Largest Health Insurance Companies of 2021," Value Penguin, Updated May 24, 2021. https://www.valuepenguin.com/largest-health-insurance-companies

45. **Here's a list the most common insurance plans:** Sarah Goodell, "Different Types of Health Plans: How they Compare," WebMD, June 15, 2020, https://www.webmd.com/health-insurance/types-of-health-insurance-plans

46. **cost averages are approximately $1,400 for individual plans and $2,800 for a family:** Healthcare.gov, "Glossary of Terms-HDHP," https://www.healthcare.gov/glossary/high-deductible-health-plan/

47. **to be in a household that is having difficulty paying medical bills:** Rachel Dolan, "High Deductible Health Plans," Health Affairs, February 4, 2016, https://www.healthaffairs.org/do/10.1377/hpb20160204.950878/full

48. **the hassle factor:** from white paper by the American Society of Internal Medicine, "The hassle factor: America's health care system strangling in red tape. American Society of Internal Medicine," 1990.

49. **Advanced payments have been referred to as subscription models:** Vivian S Lee, "Fee for service is a terrible way to pay for health care. Try a subscription model instead," Stat New, June 12, 2020, https://www.statnews.com/2020/06/12/fee-for-service-is-a-terrible-way-to-pay-for-health-care-try-a-subscription-model-instead/

50. **recent poll showed most health care professionals in the U.S. support a single-payer system:** Alicia Ault, "Majority of Healthcare Professionals Support Single-Payer System, Poll Says," Medscape, December 18, 2018, https://www.medscape.com/viewarticle/906703

51. **multiple analyses show that a single-payer system:** Christopher Cai, Jackson Runte, Isabel Ostrer, Kacey Berry, Ninez Ponce, Michael Rodriguez, Stefano Bertozzi, Justin S. White, James G.

Kahn, "Projected costs of single-payer healthcare financing in the United States: A systematic review of economic analyses," PLOS Medicine, Published: January 15, 2020, https://doi.org/10.1371/journal.pmed.1003013

Chapter 6: You Need to Ask Me First

52. **video re-enactment of a phone call with his insurance plan after suffering an acute cardiac arrest:** Taken from @DGlaucomflecken; https://twitter.com/DGlaucomflecken, Posted on July 8, 2020.

53. **GoodRx for less than $6:** "Gabapentin- Generic Neurontin," https://www.goodrx.com/gabapentin

54. **website dedicated to patient and physician stories dealing with preauths:** "Patients and Physicians Speak Out," AMA website, https://fixpriorauth.org/stories

55. **typical pre-auth form:** "Prior (Rx) Authorization Forms," eForms, https://eforms.com/prior-authorization/

56. **70% of payers say that they deny requests because what we sent over is not consistent with their guidelines:** "The Shocking Truth about Prior Authorization Process in Healthcare," ReferralMD, https://getreferralmd.com/2018/04/prior-authorization-problems-healthcare/

57. **(AACE) guidelines recommend reimaging every 3-6 months:** Melissa Young, MD, "The fight against prior authorizations," April 3, 2019, https://www.physicianspractice.com/view/fight-against-prior-authorizations

58. 83**practices spent an average of $68,274 per physician per year interacting with health plans:** "What Does It Cost Physician Practices to Interact with Health Insurance Plans?" The Commonwealth Fund, May 4, 2009, https://www.commonwealthfund.org/publications/journal-article/2009/may/what-does-it-cost-physician-practices-interact-health

59. **90% of health care leaders noted an increase in prior authorization requirements:** Claire Ernst JD, "Prior authorization

pains growing for 9/10 physician practices," MGMA Stat, September 19, 2019, https://www.mgma.com/data/data-stories/prior-authorization-pains-growing-for-9-10-physici

60. **prior authorization for prescription drugs will increase 20% per year:** "Electronic Prior Authorization- ePA National Adoption Scorecard," CoverMyMeds. http://epascorecard.covermymeds.com

61. **can cause patients to abandon their recommended course of treatment:** Andis Robeznieks, "1 in 4 doctors say prior authorization has led to a serious adverse event," AMA website, https://www.ama-assn.org/practice-management/sustainability/1-4-doctors-say-prior-authorization-has-led-serious-adverse

62. **pre-auth delays led to a serious adverse event for a patient in their care:** Andis Robeznieks, "1 in 4 Doctors Say Prior Authorization Has Led to a Serious Adverse Event," AMA website, https://www.ama-assn.org/practice-management/sustainability/1-4-doctors-say-prior-authorization-has-led-serious-adverse

63. **it cost insurers more in the long term as they seek other treatment and medication:** "The Shocking Truth about Prior Authorization Process in Healthcare," ReferralMD, https://getreferralmd.com/2018/04/prior-authorization-problems-healthcare-2/

64. **Texas is doing this now by "gold carding" physicians:** Jennifer Henderson, "Could Texas Law on Limiting Prior Authorization Delays Move the Needle Nationwide?" MedPage Today, September 21, 2021, https://www.medpagetoday.com/special-reports/exclusives/94625

65. **apply 21 principles to utilization management programs for both medical and pharmacy benefits:** "Prior Authorization and Utilization Management Reform Principles," AMA. https://www.ama-assn.org/system/files/2019-06/principles-with-signatory-page-for-slsc.pdf

Chapter 7: What's the Code for That?

66. **gathered statistical data through a system known as the London Bills of Mortality and arranged into numerical codes:**

This whole paragraph was based on "Brief History of Medical Coding," Health Information Associates, May 12, 2016, https://www.hiacode.com/education/a-brief-history-of-medical-coding/

67. **we have approximately 70,000 ICD-10 codes in health care:** "International Classification of Diseases, (ICD-10-CM/PCS) Transition – Background," Centers for Disease Control and Prevention, https://www.cdc.gov/nchs/icd/icd10cm_pcs_background.htm

68. **provides hilarious insights to the insanity of codes:** Dr. Halee Fischer-Wright, "Back to Balance," Disruption Books, Austin, TX, 2017.

69. **Struck by Orca:** Nilo Skievaski, "W56.22xA- Struck by Orca", 1st Edition, ICD-10 Illustrated, January 2014.

70. **Over 9,500 of them map to the 86 Hierarchical Condition Categories:** Stephen Gorman, "Is HCC Coding a Physician Problem?" RxRules Blog, December 12, 2019, https://www.rcxrules.com/blog/is-hcc-coding-a-physician-problem

71. **reviewers may help select codes that best reflect the provider's furnished services:** "Evaluation and Management Services Guide," CMS website, https://www.cms.gov/outreach-and-education/medicare-learning-network-mln/mlnproducts/downloads/eval-mgmt-serv-guide-icn006764.pdf

72. **Coders should code, billers should bill, and doctors should see patients:** Dr. Dike Drumond, also known as the HappyMD, wrote this in response to one of my LinkedIn post about time spent coding, His site is available at https://www.thehappymd.com

73. **Every denial costs practices $25 to $30 each to work:** The figures in this paragraph were from Tina Graham, "You might be losing thousands of dollars per month in 'unclean' claims," MGMA Insight, February 1, 2014, https://www.mgma.com/resources/revenue-cycle/you-might-be-losing-thousands-of-dollars-per-month

74. **CMS changed the documentation requirements that no longer requires a history and exam to select an E/M service:** Lisa Eramo, "E/M changes take effect January 2021," Medical Economics Journal, October 2020,

https://www.medicaleconomics.com/view/e-m-changes-take-effect-january-2021

Chapter 8: Squeeze in More Patients

75.   **How do you hide $100 from a doctor:** Dr. Toni Brayer, "How do you hide $100 from a doctor?", ACP Internist. Posted November 5, 2010.   http://blog.acpinternist.org/2010/11/how-do-you-hide-100-from-doctor.html

76.   **includes work performed for over 10,000 procedures and services covered under the CMS Physician Fee Schedule.:** CMS.gov, "Physician Fee Schedule Look-Up Tool," https://www.cms.gov/Medicare/Medicare-Fee-for-Service-Payment/PFSlookup

77.   **There are three types of RVUs:** "The Basics: Relative Value Units (RVUs)," National Health Policy Forum, January 12, 2015. https://www.nhpf.org/library/the-basics/Basics_RVUs_01-12-15.pdf

78.   **work RVU makes up around 53 percent of the total RVU across all procedures with RVU values:** Frank Cohen, "The Basics of Making RVUs Work for Your Medical Practice," Physicians Practice, July 1, 2014, https://www.physicianspractice.com/view/basics-making-rvus-work-your-medical-practice

79.   **includes these three components and a geographic adjustment factor (GAF) for each:** Frank Cohen, "The Basics of Making RVUs Work for Your Medical Practice," Physicians Practice, July 1, 2014, https://www.physicianspractice.com/view/basics-making-rvus-work-your-medical-practice

80.   **CMS pays physicians 3 to 5 times more for common procedural care than for cognitive care   :** Christine A. Sinsky, MD; David C. Dugdale, MD, "Medicare Payment for Cognitive vs Procedural Care Minding the Gap," JAMA Internal Medicine. October 14, 2013, https://jamanetwork.com/journals/jamainternalmedicine/fullarticle/1

81.   **can perform three straightforward colonoscopies with a**

polypectomy and earn 14 RVUs: Seymour Katz, MD and Gil Melmed, MD, "How Relative Value Units Undervalue the Cognitive Physician Visit: A Focus on Inflammatory Bowel Disease," Gastroenterology and Hepatology, April 2016, https://www.ncbi.nlm.nih.gov/pmc/articles/PMC4872854/

82. **health care is still 70% fee-for-service:** Tara Bannow, "Population health still at odds with fee-for-service," Modern Healthcare, April 06, 2021, https://www.modernhealthcare.com/finance/population-health-still-odds-fee-service

83. **73% of physicians prefer this model of payment:** Heather Landi, "Survey: 73 Percent of Physicians Prefer Fee-for-Service Models. Healthcare Innovation," Healthcare Innovation, October 12, 2017, https://www.hcinnovationgroup.com/policy-value-based-care/news/13029294/survey-73-percent-of-physicians-prefer-feeforservice-models

84. **physicians reported an average drop in revenue of 32% since February 2020:** Andis Robeznieks, "Physician survey details depth of pandemic's financial impact," AMA website, October 28, 2020, https://www.ama-assn.org/practice-management/sustainability/physician-survey-details-depth-pandemic-s-financial-impact

85. **few of the losers included anesthesiologists, cardiac surgeons, interventional radiologists, and thoracic surgeons:** Joyce Frieden, "2021 Medicare Fee Schedule Includes 10.2% Cut in Conversion Factor," Washington Editor, MedPage Today December 2, 2020. https://www.medpagetoday.com/practicemanagement/reimbursemel

86. **the percentage of physicians paid by a productivity-only model dropped from 51.8 percent to 42.7 percent:** Apoorva Rama, PhD, "2012-2018 Data on Physician Compensation Methods: Upswing in Compensation through the Combination of Salary and Bonus," AMA Policy Research Perspective. 2020. https://www.ama-assn.org/system/files/2020-12/data-physician-compensation-methods.pdf

Chapter 9: Charting To Infinity

87. **account quickly gained 22,000 followers and was featured in multiple publications:** @EpicEMRParody no longer exists.

88. **Larry:** Dr. Larry Slater is now a happily retired family physician. He works intermittently with my previous medical group in Santa Rosa, California.

89. **building blocks include Positive emotions, Engagement, Relationships, Meaning and Accomplishment** : Martin E.P. Seligman, "Flourish: A Visionary New Understanding of Happiness and Well-being," Free Press, New York, 2012

90. **doctors spend 5.1 hours with patients and spend 5.9 hours in the EHR** : Fred Schulte and Erika Fry, "Death by a Thousand Clicks," Fortune, March 8, 2019, https://fortune.com/longform/medical-records/

91. **Roughly 25% of that computer work happens after clinic hours:** Brian G. Arndt, John W. Beasley, Michelle D. Watkinson, Jonathan L. Temte, Wen-Jan Tuan, Christine A. Sinsky and Valerie J. Gilchrist , "Tethered to the EHR: Primary Care Physician Workload Assessment Using EHR Event Log Data and Time-Motion Observations," Annals of Family Medicine, September 2017, https://www.annfammed.org/content/15/5/419/tab-figures-data

92. **more than the United States spends treating any major class of diseases and about equal to what the country spends on public primary and secondary education instruction:** Derek A. Haas, John D. Halamka, and Michael Suk, "3 Ways to Make Electronic Health Records Less Time-Consuming for Physicians," Harvard Business Review, January 10, 2019, https://hbr.org/2019/01/3-ways-to-make-electronic-health-records-less-time-consuming-for-physicians

93. **notes in the United States are nearly 4 times longer on average than those in other countries:** N. Lance Downing, MD, David W. Bates, MD, MSc, Christopher A. Longhurst, MD, MS, "Physician Burnout in the Electronic Health Record Era: Are We Ignoring the Real Cause?" Annals of Internal Medicine, July 3, 2018m https://www.acpjournals.org/doi/10.7326/M18-0139

94. **It was an absolute nightmare. It was ridiculous, absolutely ridiculous, that we're in that circumstance:** Fred Schulte and Erika Fry, "Death by a Thousand Clicks," Kaiser Health News, March 18, 2019, https://khn.org/news/death-by-a-thousand-clicks/

95. **Physicians average 243 in-basket messages per week:** Ming Tai-Seale, Ellis C. Dillon, Yan Yang, Robert Nordgren, Ruth L. Steinberg, "Physicians' Well-Being Linked To In-Basket Messages Generated By Algorithms In Electronic Health Records," Health Affairs, July 2019, https://www.healthaffairs.org/doi/10.1377/hlthaff.2018.05509

96. **six out of 10 physicians think EHRs need a complete overhaul:** "How Doctors Feel About Electronic Health Records National Physician Poll by The Harris Poll," Stanford Medicine, 2018.

97. **shows improvements in patient care by ensuring accurate, complete, and actionable data:** . Scott Mace , "AI Can Improve Clinical Documentation, Reduce Physician Burden," HealthLeaders, April 12, 2021, https://www.healthleadersmedia.com/technology/ai-can-improve-clinical-documentation-reduce-physician-burden

98. **Interoperability and Patient Access final rule requiring the use of FHIR by a variety of CMS-regulated payers by 2021:** Fast Healthcare Interoperability Resources, Wikipedia, https://en.wikipedia.org/wiki/Fast_Healthcare_Interoperability_Res

99. **we need to standardize and reduce payer-imposed requirements:** Derek A. Haas, John D. Halamka, and Michael Suk, "3 Ways to Make Electronic Health Records Less Time-Consuming for Physicians," Harvard Business Review, January 10, 2019, https://hbr.org/2019/01/3-ways-to-make-electronic-health-records-less-time-consuming-for-physicians

Chapter 10: Let's Change What We Measure

100. **how much we spend for healthcare in the U.S. and how poorly we compare to other countries:** The bulleted items are from Roosa Tikkanen and Melinda Abrams, "U.S. Health Care from a Global Perspective, 2019: Higher Spending, Worse Outcomes?"

The Commonwealth Fund, January 30, 2020.

101. **The CMS has approximately 1,700 measures for providers within different practice settings:** Blumenthal D, Malphrus E, McGinnis JM, "Vital signs: core metrics for health and health care progress" National Academies Press, Washington (DC) 2015.

102. **you get an unsurmountable number of metrics:** Nancy E. Dunlap, David J. Ballard, Robert A. Cherry, Wm. Claiborne Dunagan, Will Ferniany, Aaron C. Hamilton, Thomas A. Owens, Terry Rusconi, Steven M. Safyer, Paula J. Santrach, Abby Sears, Michael R. Waldrum and Kathleen E. Walsh "Observations from the Field: Reporting Quality Metrics in Health Care," NAM Perspectives Discussion Paper, National Academy of Medicine, Washington, DC, 2016

103. **but most health plans use the HEDIS standard of at or below 9 percent:** Aparna Higgins, German Veselovskiy, and Lauren McKown, "Provider Performance Measures in Private and Public Programs: Achieving Meaningful Alignment With Flexibility to Innovate," Health Affairs, August 2013, https://www.healthaffairs.org/doi/full/10.1377/hlthaff.2013.0007

104. **systolic blood pressure targets for patients over sixty-five range from less than 130 mm HG to less than 150 mm Hg** : Anandita Agarwala, MD, Anurag Mehta, MD, Eugene Yang, MD, FACC, Biljana Parapid, MD, "Older Adults and Hypertension: Beyond the 2017 Guideline for Prevention, Detection, Evaluation, and Management of High Blood Pressure in Adults," American College of Cardiology, February 26, 2020, https://www.acc.org/latest-in-cardiology/articles/2020/02/26/06/24/older-adults-and-hypertension

105. **twenty-three health insurers found that they used 546 quality measures, and few of them matched across all insurers:** Aparna Higgins, German Veselovskiy, and Lauren McKown, "Provider Performance Measures in Private and Public Programs: Achieving Meaningful Alignment With Flexibility to Innovate," Health Affairs, August 2013, https://www.healthaffairs.org/doi/full/10.1377/hlthaff.2013.0007

106. **physicians and staff spent 15.1 hours per physician per week dealing with quality measures:** Lawrence P. Casalino, David Gans, Rachel Weber, Meagan Cea, Amber Tuchovsky, Tara F.

Bishop, Yesenia Miranda, Brittany A. Frankel, Kristina B. Ziehler, Meghan M. Wong, and Todd B. Evenson, "US Physician Practices Spend More Than $15.4 Billion Annually To Report Quality Measures," Health Affairs, March 2016, https://www.healthaffairs.org/doi/10.1377/hlthaff.2015.1258

107.   **compared to $34,924 for cardiology practices and $31,471 for orthopedics practices:** Lawrence P. Casalino, David Gans, Rachel Weber, Meagan Cea, Amber Tuchovsky, Tara F. Bishop, Yesenia Miranda, Brittany A. Frankel, Kristina B. Ziehler, Meghan M. Wong, and Todd B. Evenson, "US Physician Practices Spend More Than $15.4 Billion Annually To Report Quality Measures," Health Affairs, March 2016, https://www.healthaffairs.org/doi/10.1377/hlthaff.2015.1258

108.   **Despite being a $3.6 trillion annual expense:** "CMS Office of the Actuary Releases 2018 National Health Expenditures," CMS.gov Newsroom, December 5, 2019, https://www.cms.gov/newsroom/press-releases/cms-office-actuary-releases-2018-national-health-expenditures

109.   **financially penalizing acute care hospitals for the number of patients who return for a second stay within a month:** Jordan Rau, "New Round of Medicare Readmission Penalties Hits 2,583 Hospitals," Kaiser Health Network, October 1, 2019, https://khn.org/news/hospital-readmission-penalties-medicare-2583-hospitals/

110.   **observation stays for Medicare patients increased by 96 percent:** David Himmelstein Steffie Woolhandler, Quality Improvement: 'Become Good At Cheating And You Never Need To Become Good At Anything Else," Health Affairs Blog, August 27, 2015, https://www.healthaffairs.org/do/10.1377/hblog20150827.050132/f

111.   **Major teaching hospitals, which see more low income and sicker patients, were penalized more:** Sabriya Rice, "Medicare readmission penalties create quality metrics stress," Modern Healthcare, August 8, 2015, https://www.modernhealthcare.com/article/20150808/MAGAZINE/readmission-penalties-create-quality-metrics-stress

112.   **outlined key themes we should use to improve our reporting**

system: Nancy E. Dunlap, David J. Ballard, Robert A. Cherry, Wm. Claiborne Dunagan, Will Ferniany, Aaron C. Hamilton, Thomas A. Owens, Terry Rusconi, Steven M. Safyer, Paula J. Santrach, Abby Sears, Michael R. Waldrum and Kathleen E. Walsh, "Observations from the Field: Reporting Quality Metrics in Health Care," NAM Perspectives. Discussion Paper, National Academy of Medicine, Washington, DC., July 25, 2016, https://doi.org/10.31478/201607e

13. **program launched in 2012 and includes 54 specialty societies and 17 consumer groups:** All data and guidelines referenced about Choosing Wisely is located on their website at https://www.choosingwisely.org

14. **greatest way is by addressing social determinants, which make up 80-90% of a person's overall health:** Sanne Magnan, "Social Determinants of Health 101 for Health Care: Five Plus Five," National Academy of Medicine Discussion Paper, October 9, 2017, https://nam.edu/social-determinants-of-health-101-for-health-care-five-plus-five/

15. **By shifting the roughly $15 billion physicians spend reporting metrics annually to target social determinants:** Lawrence P. Casalino, David Gans, Rachel Weber, Meagan Cea, Amber Tuchovsky, Tara F. Bishop, Yesenia Miranda, Brittany A. Frankel, Kristina B. Ziehler, Meghan M. Wong, and Todd B. Evenson, "US Physician Practices Spend More Than $15.4 Billion Annually To Report Quality Measures," Health Affairs, March 2016, https://www.healthaffairs.org/doi/10.1377/hlthaff.2015.1258

16. **there are over 318,000 health apps available today, with over 200 apps being added each day:** "The Growing Value of Digital Health," IQVIA Institute Report, November 7, 2017, https://www.iqvia.com/insights/the-iqvia-institute/reports/the-growing-value-of-digital-health

Chapter 11: The Best Offense Is a Good Defense

17. **than a third of physicians (34 percent) have had a claim filed against them in their careers:** José R. Guardado, PhD, "Medical

Liability Claim Frequency Among U.S. Physicians," AMA Policy Research Perspectives, 2017.

118. **data shows that most liability claims have no merit:** Anupam B. Jena, MD, PhD, Amitabh Chandra, PhD, Darius Lakdawalla, PhD, Seth Seabury, PhD, "Outcomes of Medical Malpractice Litigation Against US Physicians,"Archives of Internal Medicine, June 11, 2012, https://jamanetwork.com/journals/jamainternalmedicine/fullarticle/1

119. **were dropped, dismissed or withdrawn:** "Data Sharing Project MPL Closed Claims 2016- 2018 Snapshot," Medical Professional Liability Association, 2019.

120. **the defendant (physician) won almost 90 percent in the case:** "Data Sharing Project MPL Closed Claims 2016- 2018 Snapshot," Medical Professional Liability Association, 2019.

121. **may take three or more years for those ending with a payment:** Seth A. Seabury, Amitabh Chandra, Darius N. Lakdawalla, and Anupam B. Jena, "On average, physicians spend nearly 11 percent of their 40-year careers with an open, unresolved malpractice claim," Health Affairs, January 2013, https://www.healthaffairs.org/doi/10.1377/hlthaff.2012.0967

122. **cost to defend a claim that eventually gets dropped or dismissed is $30,439 7:** "Data Sharing Project MPL Closed Claims 2016- 2018 Snapshot,"Medical Professional Liability Association, 2019.

123. **physicians pay over $200,000 a year in insurance premiums:** José R. Guardado, PhD, "Medical Professional Liability Insurance Premiums: An Overview of the Market from 2010 to 2019," American Medical Association Policy Research Perspectives, 2020.

124. **cost of defensive medicine per year cited vary between $46 billon and $78 billion dollars:** Paul Giancola, "Does Defensive Medicine Impact the Cost of Healthcare?" Health Law Checkup, April 5, 2017. https://www.swlaw.com/blog/health-law-checkup/2017/04/05/does-defensive-medicine-impact-the-cost-of-healthcare/

125. **Some sources the estimate is as high as $300 billion dollars:** Paul Giancola, "Does Defensive Medicine Impact the Cost of Healthcare?" Health Law Checkup, April 5, 2017. https://www.swlaw.com/blog/health-law-

checkup/2017/04/05/does-defensive-medicine-impact-the-cost-of-healthcare/

126. **to avoid the appearance of malpractice:** Emily R. Carrier, James D. Reschovsky, Michelle M. Mello, Ralph C. Mayrell, and David Katz, "Physicians' fears of malpractice lawsuits are not assuaged by tort reforms," Health Affairs, September 2010, https://www.healthaffairs.org/doi/abs/10.1377/hlthaff.2010.0135

127. **Studies show physicians may avoid inner cities:** Dennis P. Andrulis, "The Urban Health Penalty: New Dimensions and Directions in Inner-City Health Care," The National Public Health and Hospital Institute, Washington DC, 1996

128. **increasing cesarean births and decreasing overall number of deliveries:** Andrea M. Carpentieri, MA, James J. Lumalcuri, MSW, Jennie Shaw, MPH, and Gerald F. Joseph Jr, MD, "Overview of the 2015 ACOG Survey on Professional Liability," American Congress of Obstetricians and Gynecologists; 2015.

129. **planned to move to a different state because of the medical liability environment** : "2010 Illinois New Physician Workforce Study," Illinois State Medical Society, 2011, https://www.isms.org/Partners_and_Affiliates/ISMS_Resident_and

130. **State apology laws:** All the data in this paragraph comes from this reference Anna C. Mastroianni, Michelle M. Mello, Shannon Sommer, Mary Hardy, and Thomas H. Gallagher, "The Flaws In State 'Apology' And 'Disclosure' Laws Dilute Their Intended Impact On Malpractice Suits," Health Affairs, September 2010, https://www.healthaffairs.org/doi/10.1377/hlthaff.2009.0134

131. **(CANDOR) toolkit to address this issue:** "Communication and Optimal Resolution (CANDOR)," Agency for Healthcare Research and Quality, https://www.ahrq.gov/patient-safety/capacity/candor/index.html

132. **talking with colleagues after medical errors has been shown to improve physician resilience:** Yue-Yung Hu, Megan L Fix, Nathanael D Hevelone, Stuart R Lipsitz, Caprice C Greenberg, Joel S Weissman, Jo ShapiroHu, "Physicians' needs in coping with emotional stressors: the case for peer support," Archives of Surgery, March 2012, https://jamanetwork.com/journals/jamasurgery/fullarticle/1107384

133. **de-stigmatizing these services and facilitating access to them:** Margaret Plews-Ogan, Natalie May, Justine Owens, Monika Ardelt, Jo Shapiro, Sigall K Bell, "Wisdom in medicine: what helps physicians after a medical error," Academic Medicine, February 2016.

134. **while six have "total caps" that limit both economic and non-economic compensation:** Dani Alexis Ryskamp, J.D., "The Current State of State Damage Caps," Expert Institute, Updated February 12, 2021. https://www.expertinstitute.com/resources/insights/state-state-damage-caps/

135. **allowing lawyers to take up to 50% of a patient's jury award in malpractice cases:** "About the So-Called Fairness for Injured Patients Act," The Doctors Company, https://www.thedoctors.com/about-the-doctors-company/legislative-regulatory-and-judicial-advocacy/about-the-so-called-fairness-for-injured-patients-act/

American College of Medical Practice Executives (MGMA-ACMPE) with the Harwick Innovation Award and Physician Executive of the Year Award for exhibiting leadership deemed outstanding to achieve exceptional medical group performance.

When not focused on his duties as the Chief Medical Officer of a large multi-specialty medical group in California, Dr. Valenzuela channels his energy into Doc-Related, his online comic that offers a satirical look at the challenges of practicing clinical medicine through the eyes of health care professionals. His comics have been fondly referred to as "Dilbert for Health Care."

Along with his medical degree from UT Southwestern, Peter earned a master's in business administration from Auburn University. In addition, Dr. Valenzuela holds a greenbelt certificate for six sigma in healthcare from Villanova University and a healthcare innovation and entrepreneurship certificate from Duke University. Peter is also a certified trainer through The Innovator's DNA. He and his wife Vivian live in Sacramento with their cat, Zoe.

www.ingramcontent.com/pod-product-compliance
Lightning Source LLC
Chambersburg PA
CBHW080624030426
42336CB00018B/3069